*Cath*

# Link to Life

# M.E.

# Link to Life

## M.E.

**Series editor: Kevin Mulhern**

B▩XTREE

CENTRAL

First published in Great Britain in 1994 by Boxtree Limited

Text © Central Independent Television 1994

1 2 3 4 5 6 7 8 9 10

A CIP catalogue entry for this book is available from the British Library

ISBN 1 85283 9104

Cover designed by Design 23
Text designed and typeset by Wilcom Services
Printed and bound in the UK by Cox and Wyman for
Boxtree Limited
Broadwall House
21 Broadwall
London SE1 9PL

# Contents

# Preface

When the 'Link' programme first came into existence in 1976 it was thought that a series of six or twelve programmes should be enough to cover the topic of disability, but 1000 episodes later we find that there is still a mountain of material to be covered.

The central philosophy of 'Link' has been to allow disabled people to speak for themselves and raise the issues they believe are important. The topics we address have moved with the times and in the 1990s we now have an articulate disability lobby which dictates the agenda. On 'Link' today we see disabled people demanding rights not charity and also the outlawing of discrimination against them.

The significance of having a disability movement, and a television programme like 'Link' to provide a focal point for it, is to prevent disabled people feeling isolated and alone. In the past, society has treated disability as an individual catastrophe repeated six and a half million times in Britain alone. Over the years 'Link' has helped bring disabled people together to share their experiences and gain strength from each other with the aim of bringing about change.

We welcomed lending our name to the *Link to Life* series because it too gives disabled people the opportunity to tell their own stories, to explain how they live their lives and to talk about the real issues they face.

In all the years that I have been producing the 'Link' programme it has never ceased to surprise me how easy it is for disabled people to believe that they are alone and cut off and that by becoming disabled they have in some way dropped out of society and are no longer a part of it. In the mid- to late 1980s this was brought home to me very forcibly by the experience of people with M.E. (myalgic encephalomyelitis).

The 'Link' programme always has a large postbag, because disabled people and their families are often desperate for information and advice. It is often hard to predict the response we will receive to a particular programme. Anything that deals with finance or special equipment is guaranteed to get a huge amount of enquiries. However, when we broadcast our first programme on M.E. the reaction broke all records. It became clear that thousands of people are in need of help with this condition. Each time we have returned to the subject, the response has been equally overwhelming.

The fact that people are so deprived of information about M.E. indicates a number of things about the way in which people with this disorder are treated by society in general and by the medical profession in particular.

At this point a confession is in order. As the producer of the 'Link' programme I receive hundreds of ideas for programmes and during the early part of the 1980s many people suggested that I should look at the problems faced by people with M.E. I resisted, as I strongly doubted that M.E. really was a significant disabling condition. Of course, I was influenced by the prevailing medical view at the time, which treated M.E. rather like the Filofax and the mobile phone – as a symptom of being a 'Yuppie' and of having too much money and too much time on your hands. Once we had broadcast the first programme the desperation and the pain of the people who wrote in made me have considerable doubts about my initial views.

For most people M.E. is a hidden disability, so therefore there is bound to be disbelief and scepticism just as there is with conditions like epilepsy and chronic back pain, which also have no visible characteristics.

I fully recognized the depth and extent of the problem faxed by people with M.E. when someone I knew personally developed it: Mary Owens, one of the contributors to this book. In the early 1980s Mary worked with inner-city children in the Brixton and Stockwell areas of London and was one of the few people entrusted to mediate during the Brixton riots. She was, in many ways, a bit of a legend and a tireless worker with unfathomable depths of energy. When she developed M.E. the physical change in her was extraordinary. Of course she was still the same person but her energy was gone. I could see that what was happening to her was not something either psychosomatic or emotional and it certainly wasn't a case of hypochondria. She was physically weak and no matter how hard she tried, she could not regain her robust old self.

Happily many doctors are no longer as sceptical about M.E. as they were, and so the particular frustration of not being believed has diminished, although 'Link' still gets letters from people up against the same prejudice. The readers of this book will discover that M.E. is no respecter of age or status in life and can, in its most extreme form, mean that the use of a wheelchair is essential. Of course, using a wheelchair does at least banish the last vestiges of doubt about the condition.

The contributors to this book have had to change their lives and adapt to an inaccessible environment, as well as coping with a medical profession that often knows less about the condition than they do themselves. I think readers of this book will find the stories both enlightening and informative.

Kevin Mulhern
August 1994

# Paddy Masefield

Paddy is aged fifty-two and is divorced with one daughter and one granddaughter. He was a theatre director, playwright and arts consultant. He has had M.E. for eight years and for that time he has been unable to work but he sits on a number of arts, media and disability committees. He lives in Worcester.


For the first three years that I had M.E. I was obsessed with writing my story as a playwright – a playwright's portrait. But one of the results of getting M.E. was that I largely lost the ability to read and write so the portrait has changed over the last eight years as I have mellowed and re-thought the story. Like a number of people who have contracted M.E., I was extremely energetic if not hyperactive up to the time I got it. For recreation I was a marathon runner. I was directing a community play at the time, with 250 actors in Carlisle in the space of about three months. I was also commuting over the country doing some consultancy jobs, so I was leading an incredibly busy life. But it was an ideal life for me. I'd never been happier, nor in a sense freer, or able selfishly to do whatever I wanted to do in either work or leisure.

Unlike the majority of people who think they can trace their M.E. to a particular virus that they caught, I'm unable to be that specific. I did catch a cold at Lincoln Station on the way to a consultancy job that the Bishop of Lincoln had lined up. But apart from this the interesting thing is that in the very early stages I was experiencing just a slowing down, although I didn't recognize that this was what was happening to me at the time. I'd stopped running, which I hadn't fully clocked, and the standard of my work as a consultant had begun to drop. Nobody said anything to me until later, despite their mystification as to why my work had declined. I'd begun to do strange things without realizing that I couldn't account for them. For a two-mile drive, for instance, I would have to consume four bags of chocolate sweets. Like an alcoholic, I was unaware of my addiction. I'd reached a stage one day when I realized that for about a month I'd been falling asleep in the middle of each day. I used to go to great lengths to disguise it – you know, the head propped in the hand in front of a book, so as not to get caught out. I discovered one day, because somebody walked in on me, that when I was in this state it wasn't sleep but paralysis. I'd actually passed out and was totally unable to move or respond to anybody in the room. I'd been doing this quite regularly for about a month and in retrospect it was frightening to think that I was still driving a car.

This was about two months after the Lincoln Station cold. From about that time, I just ceased to function on almost every level. I was trying to write what was meant to be the most enjoyable play of my life. I'd come downstairs terribly eager to work, sit at my desk but couldn't actually see the words. I couldn't remember who the characters were that I was writing about. People told me I'd got writer's block and all the rest. I went to the doctor saying that I had problems. 'Nothing the matter,' he said. 'What you should do is take more exercise.' As my doctor was desperately overweight and I was a marathon runner, this seemed quite amusing to me at the time. I did actually listen to him though, because I was already so confused. I started going for fifteen-mile walks because of not being able to run. Often I would pass out, until one day I suddenly became a total allergic. This is a slightly dramatic state because if anybody walked into the house wearing aftershave, bang, I'd just pass out. Even a teaspoon of tap water, because of being allergic to the chlorine, would knock me out. So my life reflected the paralysis in my body, and my family, sister-in-law and brother nursed me through this state. I got progressively worse and the assumption was that I'd got something like a brain tumour and probably didn't have much longer to live.

I was given a National Health appointment for a brain scan in six month's time. As my family didn't think I was actually going to live for another six months, this introduced a rather odd relationship with the medical profession, and we started looking for private treatment. We paid for brain scans, discovered that I didn't have a brain tumour, leaving me still with the problem of not knowing what was wrong. I embarked on a series of interviews with different specialists in search of a remedy for the multiple allergies that rendered me almost paralyzed. But the allergies mystified the specialists. My family and I demonstrated to these allergy specialists that I would pass out within ten minutes of eating a slice of bread. Despite these demonstrations, the overwhelming consensus was that I was hysterical and imagining things.

The next interesting thing was that I began to meet prejudice for the first time in my life. Being middle-aged, middle-class, white and male, I'd not been exposed to anything like that before. Because I said my old profession was theatre, I was told by at least one psychiatrist in Harley Street that I was clearly as mad as a hatter because I had an overdeveloped imagination. He never thought to ask me what I **did** in theatre which was not, as a director, that dissimilar to a consultant doctor in terms of skills and demands. He assumed that I was an actor with a fortified imagination; I began to see life from an entirely new perspective before even being seriously diagnosed.

Two things eventually happened. Clare Francis came out with M.E. This is still for me the most relevant breakthrough because at that time it was a terribly brave admission to broadcast. I was one of the thousands who saw that programme. It had an immense effect on me. I burst into tears because somebody for the first time was telling me what I had. I'd recognized myself absolutely in what she said. As a result I discovered an M.E. association which provided information, including where I could find consultants capable of diagnosing it. The consultant I saw immediately diagnosed me as having M.E. But one of the slightly frightening things was that it turned out that my family had enquired about M.E. during the two years I'd been ill. At that time I had really lost my mental faculties, most of my power of speech and virtually all my power of movement. I had very little control over my own life. Other people were making decisions for me and when I was given the information on M.E., this being some seven years previously, a case as severe as mine was not recognized in the official literature. One of the things M.E. campaigners have had to fight very hard for in recent years is recognition that M.E. covers a very wide variety of situations as well as symptoms. At it's most severe, M.E. sufferers are completely bedbound, and are often without speech or movement in the body. At the other end of the spectrum they're virtually indistinguishable from so-called well people in society, except that they go to bed earlier or are unable to work long hours. There wasn't that breadth of recognition in the early literature, particularly about severity; there was nothing that said that you might have to use a wheelchair if you had severe M.E. We still have to educate and convince not only doubtful doctors but also a lot of the public. Campaigners like Clare Francis unfortunately look terribly healthy and reveal vibrant personalities when they appear on television, thus disguising the reality of M.E. behind the personality. We still have to persuade people that some of us with M.E. have immense difficulty reading and writing, need to use a wheelchair on some days, don't have the ability to dress ourselves, and so on.

Thereafter, I passed through three classic stages of disability. For the first two or three years, I was what we would now define as the medical model in that I saw my entire life through doctors, even when I got the diagnosis in negative terms. I was someone who could no longer run marathons, indeed I couldn't walk more than ten yards. I was a playwright and avid reader of books who could no longer read and write. I was incontinent. I couldn't sleep well. I couldn't focus my brain so I was intellectually impaired. I saw myself as having no role other than just staying alive to see what happened tomorrow. I literally passed each day doing jigsaw puzzles because if my brain wasn't functioning I could sit looking at one piece of jigsaw for two hours without feeling stressed. On a good day I could actually do ten pieces in an hour which was terribly exciting. But this was the nearest I got to rehabilitation.

Then I became aware of an M.E. organisation. I'd always been involved in organisations. I'd run six theatre groups in my life, so it was a natural lure for me to get involved. Like many of my colleagues I was fired up with an almost evangelistic zeal about what had happened to me during those awful two years. I wanted to write plays about how unspeakable doctors had been. I wanted to libel every doctor I'd encountered because my feelings and emotions were so affected. But here was a way of rechannelling those strong feelings. In working for this charity, I slipped into what disabled people now term 'the charitable mode'. 'Tragic but brave, former playwright, Paddy Masefield, with little-known illness, is struggling to ask charity to give him a word processor to see if we can help him learn to write again.'

The language was still fairly negative. I became a speaker for M.E. which was interesting because, as with other sufferers, M.E. affected my speech. I had all kinds of speech impediments at one stage. I was left with a very bad stammer and an inability to think quickly, so that I couldn't get even close to processing intellectually as I'm attempting to do now. But with the help of a speech therapist I was able to make public speeches and to enter debates on M.E. I attempted to travel around for a while which was fairly disastrous. I hadn't learnt how to manage my illness and would therefore bring about my own collapse nearly every time. I got involved with an M.E. organisation and became vice-chair of the M.E. Association and chair of my local groups in northern Worcestershire.

Then by accident I met someone who worked for the Arts Council of Great Britain. We talked and I said how sad it was that I couldn't do anything and that I'd more or less retired. She was bright enough to understand the context of rehabilitation and proposed that I join a committee at the Arts Council called the Arts and Disability Monitoring Committee. I said that I knew nothing about disability, but she reminded me that I had a twenty-one year knowledge of the arts which few disabled people have. This marked the beginning of a new life for me. From then on I moved in a direction which was totally new, that had no precedent in the previous forty-eight years of my life. I was meeting people whom I perceived as guru-like role models, people who had internalized something infinitely wise from which I could learn. I became a child again. One of my friends, who was writing about me in a book, said that at that time being with me was like introducing a small boy to Father Christmas. Everything was new and exciting because I had no understanding of disability, no awareness of it, and I slowly began to see myself from a totally new perspective, as a disabled person. A disabled person is not so much somebody with a negative impairment but someone disabled by a society which does not provide adequate or proper facilities. For example, if I had a wheelchair I could go to meetings without falling over and without collapsing on Paddington Station. If I got a power wheelchair I wouldn't actually need anyone to push me, I'd be independent. If I had ready access to information about disability-adapted hotels, I could in theory take myself to any part of the country, put myself to bed for two days in a hotel, get up, make an hour's speech and return to the hotel. What really changed my life – and this in many ways is now a focal point for me – was this collective sense of a family of disabled people. We are statistically an extraordinarily large group which, according to government-based statistics, is some 15 percent of society.

There are over six million of us, granting an overriding sense of belonging to a family which transcends any concept I'd previously known of nationhood, belonging to a gender or race, etc. It was a real sense of discovering a family. Some of my own close family have felt quite put out by this, as if I'd no use for them anymore. I explained that it's a new sort of family of common, shared experience which is terribly exciting and positive. For example, we share a humour on a par with Jewish humour or black humour, which I can't really share with my family because the focal point is where disability and the arts meet.

Because I'm unable to work and still have to spend three-quarters of my life lying in bed, sometimes literally in a darkened room where I can't read a newspaper or watch television, there is a great deal of time for thinking. I find time for things that I didn't have before. I found the time to join a political party and to think about what the purpose of life is in general.

I still don't know very much about my illness in medical terms. I have no idea whether my life expectancy is affected. I know some people with M.E. live to a ripe age, and it's possible I'll live to over a hundred. On the other hand, being unable to take exercise, sitting in a wheelchair, having the illness in quite a severe form, may well affect my life expectancy, and for all I know I could die if I caught a severe form of flu in five years' time. Because of this I see life differently, not as something constrained, bedbound or wheelchair-bound but as something reaffirming while it's there, so that each day becomes quite different.

A year ago, I was asked to go as a British delegate to an international conference on human rights in Helsinki, which was about minority rights in each culture. I was meeting with people from the former Yugoslavia, from Moscow, Hungary, Cyprus, who were talking about awful and terrible conditions, war, starvation and deprivation on a scale that I clearly have no experience of. But they were setting that alongside the lack of rights of a cultural minority in Finland, or of disabled people in

Britain, or of black minorities in a dominant white culture, and I found this to be an extraordinary learning experience. It was the first time I discovered, for instance, that as a disabled person dependent on State benefit as my sole source of income, I had no economic rights. The State has accepted the duty to clothe me, to feed me, to keep a roof over my head, which with an awful lot of battling has provided me, just about, with adequate means. But it has taken eight years of legal battles. It is not perceived, however, that I have the right to go to the theatre, or to travel to meet disabled people, or to want to get involved in making television programmes that change the public's perception of disability. This is not the State's problem. I started from a premise of no economic rights and no economic freedom. I'm still dependent on a society that sees things in terms of medicine and charity. But I now have a focus that in a way seems much more important than what I was trying to do in the theatre – I can even contribute to a change in disability issues (having, for instance, written the end of Brian Rix's maiden speech in the House of Lords on disability, and contributed the story that he used there), through to the much more general point of wanting to change the perception of people with disability through television. I'm a member of Central Television's Regional Advisory Council, which I fought terribly hard to get, because Central will now allow me to make presentations to them concerning disability. This actually gives me a route which I can't get through paid employment to try to change the nature of society.

In retrospect, those early days of M.E. are still a bit of a haze. One of the dominant symptoms was the lack of short-term memory. While with great effort I can recall nearly all events before M.E., for quite large areas of my life since then, memories are blotted out. It was extremely difficult for me at that time to write more than half a dozen lines. Focusing was a big problem. Because I couldn't read, people gave me tapes of books and radio programmes. I couldn't understand why I derived no enjoyment from these and just switched them off after five minutes. Having no short-term memory, I couldn't remember who the characters were so I had no interest in a plot because I wasn't held by it. This had its obvious comic sides which we used to share in M.E. support groups. At night you might put a pound of butter on the doorstep and try to put the cat in the fridge because of being confused about what you did with different things. One example that stands out in my memory is when I went into the toilet, but not having the foggiest idea what I was doing in there, I reemerged five minutes later needing to go to the toilet. However I could open the fridge door feeling hungry, open it and look for something to read in the fridge.

When I was really at my worst, I lost virtually all my power of speech. I subsequently discovered that I was hyperventilating dramatically, which was screwing up my speech and left me with a very severe stammer. Again there was no medical rehabilitation provided so I had to get hold of a speech therapist myself. She put me through a range of tests which don't even exist in this country (they're from America) to establish my intellectual powers of reasoning as well as speech, on the sort of scale that might be used in this country with people who have had a stroke or a car crash. According to these tests, I showed up on a scale of around five out of ten, a considerable degree of intellectual impairment. I couldn't pair up words, I couldn't understand opposites – black and white, say – and my concentration span diminished after ten or fifteen minutes, so I often become argumentative.

Movement was desperately limited. M.E. is often wrongly described in terms of lack of energy or exhaustion. I would say it's about very impaired mobility. Because I'd been a marathon runner and a keep-fit freak, I used to get out of bed and attempt to do press-ups. The family was keen that I should get fresh air and I was also encouraged to walk around the house in the afternoon. It would take an hour and a half to cover a distance of 100 yards, having to sit down maybe ten or fifteen times during that period. I was a total allergic, which meant that I would pass out on contact with any allergen. I was put on all sorts of weird diets and I lost about four stone in weight.

All my symptoms are partly connected with the allergies which could induce total paralysis. I have partial problems of numbness, have become extremely clumsy, and when I am able to walk, I walk with sticks because I have such poor balance. I have walked into doorways and smashed virtually every plate in the house through being unable to tell where either the table or the plate was. I have individual symptoms which can be quite distressing when you've got no medical authority or reference point telling you why or what. The fact that you have pain in all your joints or muscular twitches all over the body can be more distressing than having great pain or an absolute splitting headache. Just to get through a day means dependence on pain killers, resulting in very severe stomach malfunction. To begin with I lived with a permanent stomach ache, and would have to be no more than thirty seconds from a toilet. The prevailing feeling was that my body had gone bad on me, like something left in the fridge for too long. I had no facility to be objective or explain things as I can now. It would be a hard enough struggle to say 'It's like your brain being filled with porridge' – which wouldn't mean much to people, so I'd say 'Well, try and imagine you've got the worst hangover you've ever had, you've got a really bad bout of flu, you've got a migraine and you've just run fifteen miles in that condition...'. And that still wouldn't be a really adequate description. For about two years it became an obsession to try and find a way of properly describing the condition, because all of us who had M.E. felt the same. Very often our closest family and friends actually had no idea what it felt like. Many people with M.E., talking to me through the network of M.E. support groups, often state that the most distressing thing of all that is that their closest family, partners, parents, children – even sometimes after ten years – have so little understanding that they'd still turn up at Christmas saying, 'Why don't you go on holiday'? or 'Why don't you get the car out?'

The greatest compliment my enemies probably pay me is to say I'm a defender of lost causes. I think 'fighting for lost causes' is immensely valuable. But whether anybody else perceives disability or the problem of getting proper recognition for M.E. as a lost cause, clearly I don't. I have wanted to write plays about issues, to be a fighter. The fighting instinct is there even to the extent that at my very lowest, when I had no physical movement and doctors were being really dismissive and rude to me, I can remember wanting to hit them. I would normally call myself a pacifist so this was a new and strange reaction. Fortunately nobody knew, because all that actually happened was that my fingers twitched a little.

We don't know the exact statistics in terms of disability affecting attitude because it constantly comes back to this lack of an epidemiological study, no statistical base. But from swapping experiences and observations, it would appear that possibly more than 50 percent of people who get M.E. also get a form of clinical depression. I happen to be in the lucky 40 percent or whatever who don't have that depressive element; I've managed to maintain a sense of humour even at my lowest ebb. I can remember falling over on a dog that was trying to help push me on because I'd come to a standstill and finding it all terribly funny, while not knowing who my best friend was on the telephone strikes me as amusing rather than depressing, so I really am one of the lucky ones.

Life experience as a result of having M.E. has taken on a transitional move from negative to positive. First of all, like most people who have become ill and particularly like most people who can't get a diagnosis for their illness, I was terribly sad about the things I couldn't do. I had a job and a way of life as a theatre director and as one of the country's leading arts consultants that was wonderful. People would suggest that I'd fallen ill for hypochondriacal reasons because I couldn't cope with life. I persevered by saying that life is wonderful, it's filled with humour and meeting people, and being able to write plays. This doesn't mean that there wasn't a great sense of loss. Counsellors whom I've met subsequently have actually said that the transition was probably like a bereavement. One of the strongest manifestations of this concerned the Malvern Hills. When I worked on Sundays in Worcester, I would run from one end of the Malvern to the other and back again, no matter what the weather. Being deprived of doing this hit me so severely that even if I looked at the Malverns I burst into tears.

There were other very significant losses which again are very like bereavement or passing through divorce or family break-up. I lost nearly all the friends I had before M.E. either because they couldn't cope with the change in me or couldn't cope with someone so severely ill, or just because their lives took them elsewhere. I was confined to a single room in a single house so there was an immense overall sense of deprivation, loss, of feeling very alone because the world didn't understand me. The inability to handle stress caused by M.E. can make you very erratic in personality. Your mood swings violently when under great pressure, and there's a tendency to have panic attacks. I remember trying to get out of the house because I thought it would be healthy to take some exercise. Within 100 yards of hobbling along on two sticks, I was lying under a hedge curled up in a foetal position, crying in terror of the open road ahead of me.

The redeeming and positive aspects of having developed this illness are that my friends and family now share a joke and say in my presence that disability is the best career move I ever made. This has nothing whatever to do with hypochondria or it being a wonderful life to be confined to your bed dependent on state benefit, rather it has to do with the fact that I have found a sense of purpose, a sense of relationship to the world and a sense of family. Some people find it through supporting a football team, I found it through sharing with disabled people. It is not about five cripples getting together and sharing their hatred of the world, but about the fact that disability has put me in close contact with people of opposite gender, closer than I'd probably experienced even being a father of a daughter or being married twice. My feeling of understanding the world and friendships transcends age. Some of the wisest people I know are half my age but may have been disabled all their lives. Meeting people who have faced prejudice, who have understood and lived through oppression, who have come through these experiences with positive virtues, is incredibly uplifting. People come into my house and may find it pretentious that Nelson Mandela's picture is on the wall, or that I sometimes wear an ANC badge. Yet I see people who come through oppression as quite extraordinary, and infinitely wiser, compassionate and sensitive. The plight of Nelson Mandela, of all that wisdom being locked up for twenty-seven years, is not far from the plight my colleagues and M.E. associates share. I've used the analogy that people with M.E. are in some ways – and this was an analogy that got me into trouble – like the Beirut hostages who were locked up in a small space and suffered sensory deprivation, deprived of reading materials, or food and light. I find it very interesting that many of those hostages, who suffered unspeakable things, perhaps even physical torture, have nonetheless emerged as wiser people, or as people with a capacity to speak for other human experiences. I now have a feeling that I belong more in the world, that I know a little bit more about the world and its shortcomings set in ignorance. I was born in Uganda in a multiracial country. I've always been concerned with issues of racism and cultural diversity and I thought I had an understanding of what it was like to be black although I was white. One of the things that disability has taught me is that it's terribly difficult as well as presumptious to actually know what somebody else's experience is like unless you've been through it yourself. I suppose the most exciting thing is that most people coming into their fifties don't feel as I do as if they're just starting at school or university, that life is an open book and each day is a learning experience. There is a sense in which my life is getting fuller and more exciting daily, and yet I have spent most of the last month in bed because I have just had an M.E. relapse. I've been unable to keep appointments outside the house. I've been unable to make important speeches which I struggle to put on to tape and send to London conferences in my absence. There's no way I'm kidding myself that I don't still have an ongoing, and probably a lifetime illness, as well as being a disabled person. Even so, what's much more exciting to me is what I can see.

It appalls me that the medical profession is still so ignorant and arrogant. It's difficult to understand why doctors should have the status they have when they shut themselves off to M.E. We should assume that they are no wiser than playwrights, poets or politicians who are powerful human beings but who only occasionally get things right.

M.E. has made me realize that society is an incredibly oppressive place for disabled people. You have to go through the personal experience of going in a power wheelchair into a supermarket and being showered with four-lettered abuse by middle-aged shoppers in a hurry who trip up over your wheelchair and resent you being in their space. It's been an extraordinary shock to meet British Rail employees who, as part of their job, have to push my old National Health Service wheelchair at Oxford Station to get me from one platform to another, across the lines and up the other side. It's quite horrific when the person assigned to you asks how long you've been in a wheelchair (on this particular occasion, six years), and on hearing responds, 'Good God, if I'd been a burden on society that long I'd have shot myself'. This was the contribution I made to Lord Rix's speech, a metaphor for the resentment people feel. When you're sitting in a wheelchair people won't meet your eyes, they don't know how to behave towards you; sometimes travelling on a train I'm patronized by people who treat me almost as if I was a three-year-old. It's an eye-opener when it comes to what little awareness society has about any of the redeeming positive features of disability. I know my colleagues as disabled people who are also artists, wise people, politicians, mothers or friends. In society disability it seems is a label that you're lumbered with. The label means that you forfeit your identity so that you are seen only in terms of the label and not in the functioning role you might have in society. For me it's become a massive campaign for civil rights.

I have a growing collection of British Rail anecdotes which merge together to make a black comedy. Life is littered with daily humour, and this was particularly true when my M.E. was slightly more severe, because I lost control of the English language. Opposites creep in, so one literally says John when one means Jill, or black when one means white. Sometimes I'd be saying the exact opposite of what I'd meant and wonder why my companions would fall about laughing. You're incapable of monitoring what you are saying as your brain is so fuzzy. Life was an on-going series of jokes. The business of getting a pound of butter out and trying to read it, or wondering which part of the book you ate if you were hungry is both tragic and comical. Artists have struggled to reflect this on canvas. Those of us who write plays try to use a dramatic form to capture the absurdity so true to life.

There is actually very little that I'm doing for the first time because of being part of a movement. There is a great sense of pride in contributing to television programmes through the Central Television committee, trying to increase employment for disabled people in the arts industry. The latter is something I've been involved in first with Lord Rix and then Lord Snowdon for the last two years. The concept that lives will not be as wasted in the future is very important to me. I had a wonderful life in the theatre up to the age of about forty-five, but it's a very average career for a person of my age and background. What really shocks me is that there is no person in the whole country, disabled from birth, who is allowed the same experience. This says something horrendous about the legal, employment and economic oppression of disabled people. This is why campaigning in that area is vital; convincing just one more employer that they ought to fulfil the 1944 Employment Act with their 3 percent quota is a real achievement. If I'd not been allowed to do those things that I had fun doing, I think my life would have been wasted. If other disabled people are deprived, surely it is a waste of their lives. My sense of achievement mainly concerns politics, employment, and education. I'm very proud of trying to do my bit within the M.E. movement to change awareness and perception of M.E. by talking about it on radio, on television, in books. I've been forthcoming because a lot of people with M.E. are reluctant to be.

Disability has almost helped me into the first stages of maturity. Like many human beings heading towards fifty, I'm still the same immature adolescent that I was at twelve, still feeling an idiot and a buffoon, and I think the experience of disability has given me more time. It's given me more time to get to know my family, to understand some of the things that happened within my family, which I was always too busy to do before.

I've come to feel a sense of achievement about quite small things. Despite the loss of reading and writing, despite the lack of concentration span, I've realized that what's more important is actually being aware of what's happening in the entire world, having a genuine concern rather than being very self-centred as so many of us are, particularly in theatre. I think my sense of achievement is to do with private things, in realizing that I need to learn a great deal of wisdom from other people.

In general I've been very slow to really fully manage my illness. If I was running a complex organisation like a theatre and it took me eight years to understand how to run it, I'd be kicked out of the job probably within the first two months. It's fairly extraordinary to me that I only realized, after seven years of illness, that if I applied to the council for a 100 percent grant for £5,000 to install a stairlift in my house, it would mean I would have more mental energy than physical energy as a result of not trying to walk up and down my stairs twice a day. I only enquired about a power wheelchair a year ago because a disabled colleague asked what on earth I was doing with a manually operated one? It just hadn't occurred to me. In the last year, with the help of friends and family, I've acquired a fax, an answerphone, a video recorder and even a satellite dish, because these things enable me to manage my life, help me to stay involved with events and to maintain contact with people in a way that I couldn't otherwise achieve if I was confined to bed.

The most important solution to problems for me has been in beginning to understand how to manage my illness and accepting that I have more to offer the world and am less dependent on other people. Other problems solved are to do with mobility and the perception that if you put the same degree of planning (very common for most disabled people) into a journey as you do in taking part in something as simple as a conference, then you can do almost anything.

Other problems remain unresolved because most of them are the big issues of wanting changes in legislation, of wanting people who sit in Parliament to be aware of my condition and to take me seriously. I'm proud of the fact that along with two colleagues in Worcester, we have managed to get our local Tory MP extremely interested in M.E. matters to the extent that we've asked him to be a patron of the group. It's some achievement that he's asked half a dozen questions in the house and has written to ministers repeatedly about M.E. If we had that impact all over the country we could really bring about legislative change in the state benefits and for the medical appraisal of M.E.

The other serious unresolved problem is the discrimination that M.E. sufferers continuously encounter. Discrimination is rife because a lot of people with M.E. have no outward signs of illness. We can look ordinarily healthy and if we don't need sticks or wheelchairs to get us about, then despite a hundred yards being the maximum mobility, there is no badge that signifies an ill or disabled person. There is this prevailing prejudice and discrimination because the public can't spot the illness as they might, say, with chicken pox or a broken leg. Many believe it's a hypochondriac state, and I hear people I've now known for several years say, 'I think I now understand the illness a little bit better because I've seen you for four years, but I have to say when I first met you I thought you were a phoney.' This attitude is very tough, particularly on youngsters. It's a constant problem for all of us involved in M.E. campaigning, making provision for school-age children with M.E. Even though the State is obliged to provide home tuition if you are unable to go to school and has to accommodate you within a school no matter what your circumstances, most young people with M.E. are being deprived of a proper education.

There are levels of discrimination too within the medical profession, in terms of the area of benefits you don't qualify for. Benefits are designed for people who are medical models, those who have lost limbs or with impaired faculties, the blind or the lame, etc. There is very little benefit provided for those who are actually *ill*, so as a result there is immense discrimination in legal, medical and benefit terms. A person with M.E., particularly when they first get it, probably feels like a leper did 100 years ago.

Three months ago my family came to visit me. My granddaughter loves swimming, but because I was allergic to chlorine, going anywhere near a swimming pool would make me pass out. My allergies have improved under treatment over an eight-year period, which is another enormous step. I was taken to a swimming pool which accommodates a wheelchair. Having put on weight as a result of being unable to take exercise, I found that I floated quite well, and I can't describe to you the excitement of finding that I was floating in a swimming pool, a feat I never thought I'd manage again. It was still a knife edge though because of the terror at the prospect that I might pass out if I came into contact with the chlorine.

Although it's now eight years since I last worked, I acquired an ambition two years ago which I identified as my first professional ambition since having M.E. I wanted to make a career change into the media. When I left university I wanted to be a television director but wasn't accepted, and became a theatre director instead. I was immensely happy, but on approaching fifty, I decided to try again to get into television. Because I can't work, I'm limited in terms of the time I can offer. Nonetheless since making that decision I've managed to get on the regional board of Central Television; I'm a member of two British Film Institute committees; and I now chair an editorial board currently overseeing a book about past, present and future images of disability on television and cinema. As I become more and more involved with the world of television, I realize how good it has been and lucky for me to be able to make a new career move in middle age.

On the other hand, the sense of failure that I have is very severe in that my life is so self-centred. I've not actually found time or the skills to organize a social life. As a slightly wiser human being than I was twenty years ago I can see that not having 'switch-off' time, a social life, a wider range of friends who aren't just professional, is actually a failure. For the first time now I'm learning to make more time for a granddaughter and a daughter. But my real success will be if in ten year's time I've also found a way of doing normal things like going out to dinner with someone. These are the things that I haven't yet achieved.

In the early days I found that panic attacks rendered me dysfunctional. I still have a terror of being unable to travel any distance or to take part in something. I haven't yet beaten sound sensitivity. I am sound and light sensitive, like a number of people with M.E., which means that I can't cope with public places. I would love to be able to go to a pub, for example, but if you've got M.E. you are not allowed to drink alcohol because of the negative effect it has. There have been times when someone did try to take me in a wheelchair to a pub on a sunny summer's day but within a short period of time I discovered that there is no way I can cope with the noise. There have been occasions at public meetings where if two discussion groups are going on in the same room, I have to say to colleagues that I can't cope. If there is more than one sound I cannot separate them. If two other people are having a conversation on the other side of the room I couldn't have a separate conversation with someone in the same room because I'd get confused over who was talking to me.

I regret that I'm never going to run the marathon again. There are also a couple of other things that I would desperately like to do that are terribly important to me but which I'm not sure if I ever will be able to do. I was a playwright, a jobbing playwright, a technician playwright but an experienced one. I've had something like thirty plays performed and I've collaborated with people whom I've thought were the genius half, where I've provided the this-is-how-we-turn-it-into-a-play half. I'm not underestimating my part, I'm just thinking in terms of skill, like being more of a mechanic rather than the driver. Since I have had M.E., I've discovered that thing that all playwrights long to have which is a voice. It's a voice which expresses the black humour of disability, of M.E. Because I have such difficulty reading and writing and because I have memory difficulties and co-ordination difficulties, I've not found a way yet of writing a play. Some people have suggested that I should process it through interviews. I have friends who are much more severely impaired than I am, like the journalist and television writer, Chris Davies, who has suggested we write a play together. He has cerebral palsy and yet still manages to be a writer, so he sees my impairments as terribly modest in comparison. My burning ambition is to return to being a writer and to say things that are more important than anything I have said in the past. But I am also up against a considerable fear of failure which is a massive hurdle to jump.

At exactly the time that I got M.E., my daughter, who would have been about seventeen at the time, set off around the world. When she came back into my life, she'd grown into an infinitely wise person, and so we built a completely new relationship in which she gradually came to understand an immense amount about M.E., and in a way became my best friend and the person to whom I usually turn if I'm severely ill. She is the person I ring up and say I'm feeling awful, I've got nothing intelligent to say, just talk to me for five minutes to cheer me up.

The relationship with my parents is curious, because when I fell ill, aged about forty-five, they were elderly and in their late seventies. In the past I'd often travel an hour's journey to where they live down the motorway to chop wood for them and do some gardening. In the first two or three years that I was ill they suddenly and unexpectedly had to revert to their previous parenting roles because I had no partner and the State didn't pick me up. It was in a sense my parents, and then through them a sister-in-law who had been a nurse, and an older brother, who literally gave me a home and looked after me. I owe a great deal to them.

Friends are a difficult factor. Most of the friends I had were related to my work and my profession. I was one of those people who had a number of acquaintances, colleagues, people I liked, but – I guess like many men – few very close friends. When I fell ill, most of my friends, because of the ignorance surrounding M.E., couldn't cope. It was the time that we first began to become aware of AIDS, and because of prejudice regarding people who work in the theatre and because I got very thin as a result of my allergies, I think an awful lot of people assumed I'd got AIDS. A number of people thought I'd had a nervous breakdown and couldn't handle that because they wanted to tell me to pull myself together. At one stage I experienced a great sense of loss – we come back to the word bereavement – it felt as though I didn't have any friends any more. Throwing myself into M.E. support groups was an obvious way of building new friendships. These are people who might have limited energies, they might have very limited emotions to spare, but they have an incomparable understanding because they too have M.E. I would say that even people I don't meet very often who are disabled are closer than friends from the past whom I might have known for ten years or more. I have acquired a new set of friends along with a new set of values and a new set of eyes.

My whole situation re employment and the financial implications is probably unusual because at the time I fell ill I was self-employed. I was either engaged as a freelance theatre director where you're immediately thrown into a very close working relationship with people, or I'd work as a playwright which might mean sitting in my room for three months writing before sharing it with several hundred people. I was also working as an arts consultant which would mean trips to Barrow-in-Furness or Great Yarmouth or St Helens, to work on my own. When I fell ill I had no employers, no one had any obligations to me, so all sources of income ceased. I had no contracts that covered illness – all my contracts were dependent on my being able to do the work – and I had no pension rights. Because I'd chosen to work all my life in the arts, putting on low budget community plays, I had no savings. The first situation that had a great impact was during the first year that I was ill when I was literally receiving something like £25 a week from the State. While I waited to be diagnosed and to qualify for benefit, I started to lose all my possessions: my car went and so did other things that I could sell. My greatest worry was that it would be necessary to sell my house. I was literally supported for my first two years – an extraordinary thing for me to have forgotten until now – by colleagues, many of whom I didn't know very well, in an organisation called The Director's Guild of Great Britain. Although I had been one of the founding members, I was a rather obscure kind of country member, who had sat on their council. They created a public fund that they advertised through performances and raised £3,000 to keep me financially secure for the first two years. It was my family who looked after my health and my professional colleagues who looked after my finances.

I've never been denied ordinary medical treatment but I had to have some specialist medical treatment privately because the State denies that. It's interesting that the allergy treatment that worked for me and for some of my colleagues used to be available on the NHS fifteen years ago. It was one of the earliest cuts of the Thatcher government years, and so the doctors who practised this line of research and treatment have had to do it privately. My family have had to pay for it.

The only alternative treatment that's been an incredible help, and I'm now dependent on it every day, is hypnotherapy. About eight years before I got M.E. I was nearing a classic mid-life crisis. I was approaching forty, my second marriage had broken down, I was very overweight, I drank very heavily and I smoked the best part of eighty cigarettes a day – not a very healthy state for a thirty-eight year old. Then because of a sense of impending crisis, I got myself roughly into shape. I found a hypnotist who cured me of my worst vices in the space of three weeks. I never want to smoke another cigarette in my life. I became teetotal. I lost weight from running and subsequently turned into an addictive marathon runner and keep-fit freak. Thus because I'd had such a positive earlier experience under hypnosis, when I found myself falling prey to panic attacks as part of M.E., I started hypnotherapy. It was after six one-hour sessions that the panic attacks stopped and I came away with a tape from the hypnotherapist that I use every day. This enables me to manage with the resources I have. I know that I cannot make myself well through hypnosis. Though I tell myself that I will get well, that I will be able to run or whatever, it doesn't really work like that. Yet what you can do is quite extraordinary. M.E. can make one very garrulous – it's one of the symptoms – and if I'm going to a committee meeting, particularly if I'm chairing, it's not in one's best interest to behave like that. So under self-hypnosis I can say, 'You will be very aware of other people, you will enjoy being quiet because this enables you to benefit from other people's wisdom,' and so on. I have now acquired, as a result of the experience of three or four different hypnotists, the ability to give myself a very mild self-hypnosis; it's not much more than what other people might derive from yoga or other techniques, which induce a deep state of relaxation. Sadly when I have a relapse, that is, when I become more ill than my normal state, I can't use this aid because of the severity of the illness. With the loss of mental faculties I am unable either to hypnotize myself or to be hypnotized by the tape.

I gave up driving a car because I caught myself one day doing a U-turn while having a panic attack on a dual carriageway. I didn't have a clue about what I was doing. I realized then that I was totally unsafe on the road. There are people with M.E. who can drive occasionally, but clearly I couldn't. As a result I lost the independence I'd taken for granted for twenty years. Now, however, as far as I am concerned, the use of a wheelchair is equivalent to using a car and is no less dignified a form of practical transportation. In considering a visit to Birmingham, you wouldn't dream of doing it on foot, you would go by car or by train. If you can accept that you can't walk fifty miles, and this fact isn't a hindrance and doesn't diminish your sense of dignity, why is it that other people cannot accept it? Having a wheelchair means that, provided the road surface is reasonable, I can go for a walk with my daughter and granddaughter or anybody.

But transportation requires immense planning and is potentially very depressing. The train journey to London in itself obliges me to go to bed for sixteen hours beforehand or I'd be seriously unwell. An Intercity train only has two wheelchair spaces, and, until very recently, those spaces were not built with access to a toilet, which meant that it wasn't feasible to be in a wheelchair and also to make use of the toilet. If on the day I want to go to London two other people in wheelchairs also want to go, one of us would have to travel in the guard's van because there are only two spaces. Sometimes staff don't turn up, or the computer that alerts them to my arrival in a wheelchair breaks down.

As a middle-aged man I became terribly house-proud, which I never was when I was married. When I first got M.E., I used to worry desperately about the fact that I couldn't do the dusting or the ironing. When, with the help of a lot of friends and colleagues, home-care help was organised for me (which I'm still dependent on), I used to get terribly concerned that other people would not clean my house to the standard I had maintained. It's taken me a very long time to appreciate that the state of one's house is not a priority.

About six weeks ago I attempted for the first time in four years and in a state of crisis, to iron a shirt which I think was probably what triggered the subsequent month's relapse. I don't have the muscular power to lift or repeat actions so I have to pay someone to do the housework. The system of home-care support has been incredibly good in my experience. Individuals provide a very good level of care and support. But the decline of economic resources, cuts to the social services, and so on, has meant people losing benefits such as housework, ironing, and bathing people. The outcome of this in most cases has been seriously debilitating. I, for example, am about 50 percent worse off now than I was six years ago.

When I was severely ill and returned to my own house, I was clearly unable to cope, anybody could see this, and I was still repeatedly passing out. I think I got the best out of the social services. I couldn't get to a destination to receive my benefit, or to fill in forms. I couldn't take a postal order or giro to the post office so they had to come to me, which resulted in the social services making some very simple assessments. They offered to have a second telephone line installed beside my bed and to pay the rental for it. This literally was a lifeline because I was dependent on the goodwill of one set of neighbours whom I would call and get them to ring for an ambulance.

I have recently been provided with a door-opening device both in my bedroom and in the kitchen. Also, through the occupational therapist I got a stairlift installed, so there are now a number of essential aids. Discovering small supplementary tools, like magnifying glasses to help me read, or elastic shoelaces to help me overcome the fact that I can't easily reach my shoes, have created other lifelines that I should have been plugged into when I was most severely ill and impaired. These are things that I've learnt very late in the process, because we are all amateurs when we first meet illness or disability; we haven't had the training.

The sort of thing I can really do without is being patronized. For example, if I'm in a wheelchair and with someone who's not in a wheelchair, people will speak to the person who's behind the wheelchair. The most bizarre instance was when my daughter and her partner, who are both very athletic and tough, decided one New Year's Day that they would try and get me to the top of the Malverns in my wheelchair. It was pouring with rain and I was almost sobbing, afraid that I'd catch pneumonia. They wrapped me up in three mackintoshes and because the ground was muddy they had to carry me up in the wheelchair. We got half way up the Malverns and met a number of hardy people exercising their dogs, all of whom bestowed a patronizing little smile on me and then turned to my family and said, 'How nice that you've brought him up'. When I lost the power of speech I knew I couldn't speak, but I sometimes wanted to provide an answer to a simple question. If somebody said 'Would you like a cup of tea?' my brain couldn't produce the word yes, or a thumb up or a nod or anything, so I'd look to the questioner like a vegetable, although I knew inside myself that I was still a person. But what really got to me was that anyone perceiving me as a disabled person automatically made prejudicial assumptions.

Emotionally, it's been up and down. I've now met several thousand people with M.E. and I know that when you are having a bad time with it you cannot handle any stress. This is not psychological but a biological fact, which is connected to what's called the fight and flight mechanism. All human beings have this. If someone suddenly mugs you or you are about to be attacked by a lion, you will find that you can run three times as fast or as far as you normally can. The body is designed to pump up adrenalin levels given threatening situations. When you've got M.E. it seems to me that you are permanently drawing on that fight or flight reflex in order to stimulate energy. There are therefore no spare reserves for stress. A pointless argument would within five minutes reduce me to a state of uncontrollable rage. I once found myself attacking my aged parents physically, just because they'd suggested a change in my diet. This resulted in my raving for three hours, screaming and shouting, and trying to tear up bits of the lawn, which was as terrifying an experience for me as it was for them. Learning to live with that in a manageable way made me realize that in those early days of M.E., I lost my temper with people in a way that was not normal.

I was shocked to discover when I first fell ill, how little I knew about the benefit system. I had little entitlement, partly because I had a very small amount of savings and I was expected to use these resources first while the system contributed nothing. I became poorer and poorer to such an extent that I could no longer afford to live in my house. Then, in either 1985 or very early 1986, a benefit assessment officer saw that I clearly needed an additional heating allowance and a daily home help, so social services awarded me these benefits because my economic situation was so desperate. I was living on a variety of extremely weird diets which I believed were keeping me alive and I got a £50 diet allowance a week. In 1985/86, I received approximately £125 per week from income support, which amounted to invalidity benefit, income support, special diet allowance, an allowance to pay for a cleaner, and a heating allowance. For many people, £125 per week in 1985 seemed a lot of money and indeed I could live on that sum, given that I'd stopped smoking, didn't drink, and wasn't taking holidays or going out much.

But in April 1986 legislation was introduced that halved those benefits. Diet benefit, cleaner benefit, extra heating benefit were all cut. If you take real inflationary figures – and there was high inflation in the late 1980s – I now receive as my legal entitlement approximately 50 percent of what I received six years ago. Some of my physical states like mobility have worsened, so there is no logic in receiving less money. In order even to maintain that 50 percent I have had to fight the benefit system continuously. I've had to appeal, and without a right to legal aid. Because I can't afford a solicitor I tried going to a free self-help agency but it turned out to be absolutely useless. So each April, when my benefit was decreased I managed, with immense difficulty and considerable pain, to write a one-sided letter protesting against the immoral negligence I was experiencing. I said I would be contacting my MP and that I would personally see to it that television plays would be written and broadcast revealing these injustices. In most cases, within a month, I would get my benefit restored and the cut would be withdrawn. Apart from maybe one occasion, no explanation was ever given to me for the sudden renewal of my benefit. One was just left with this feeling that by being stroppy and refusing to be fobbed off, you would finally get what you were entitled to. But if you lie down and submissively give in to the instinct that tells you not to make a fuss, it's guaranteed you'll get trampled on by the system.

I feel angry about a government which, while publicly proclaiming that it has increased benefit, has after all that fighting still cut my funds by 50 percent. When I talk about the need for legislation to underline everything connected not only with disability but also very specifically with M.E., it's because all the new government legislation due to be passed this April, which introduces new words like incapacity benefit, threatens to make it four times as difficult to get benefit for the condition of M.E.

It is always pointed out that M.E. exists and is recognized in law because Edwina Currie as Junior Health Minister actually got it put into the statute books back in 1986 or 1987. In reality though, it doesn't exist, in that as yet no one has funded an epidemiological study. The first issue I would want to resolve is that legal recognition of an illness or medical condition is only possible through an appropriate way of responding to that condition. That is, appropriately responding to it with benefits, welfare, education, and a charter of rights. If you can actually define what the illness is, what the range of symptoms are, and what the incidence is in different parts of the country, in gender, in age and so on, you have a basis for arguing a case. In order to change legislation, we first of all need an epidemiological study. The government will never put up the money for this and no voluntary charity is ever going to be able to do a nationwide study that will take several years to complete. However, if that study is a right in law, if those that are arguing can get that established, we then have a basis on which we can begin to educate doctors who at the moment are at liberty to dispute that this condition exists. It's necessary to have clear statistical proof, together with an explanation of what M.E. looks like and how to recognize it, provided by government agencies. Medical charities do this at the moment – the M.E. Association and Action for M.E. provide excellent advice for GPs – but this doesn't have the force that it would have if it came from HM Chief Medical Officer and from the Establishment.

It's not even research initially, it's just a recognition of the facts. Like almost any group of people who feel oppressed or marginalized, we are merely asking to be put on the same playing field as everyone else by recognizing the facts. If you've got facts you can then go on to argue that in traditional medical training this is a complex condition to recognize or diagnose, so doctors need to acquaint themselves with the symptoms of M.E. In effect this is what they do each year with a wide variety of 'new illnesses' or conditions. We know more through the medical profession updating itself. With that principal accepted as a premise to work on, we can begin to find a whole raft of rights regarding benefits, work, education. Even a government with which I may choose to disagree is able to recognize that if you've lost the function of two limbs, it is unlikely that you will be able to compete in a marathon, and that using a wheelchair to compensate for the loss of your legs is a straightforward, logical step.

As I've said, because of my lack of muscular power and co-ordination, I cannot do any complex cooking. Not only can I not physically do it, it's dangerous, I throw things over myself that can scald me and so on. The campaign to get this recognized as a hazardous way of existing and for help with the cooking to be provided, has been a momentous battle against bureaucracy. Once a year at least, sometimes two or three times, I have to fill in forty- to fifty-page forms in which other people have to verify that I am not lying.

Even more than new legislation, I want basic recognition of the same rights that are normal for all human beings; that if you go to a doctor with this condition called M.E., you will not be mocked or scorned. I've known of a case where, aged thirty, someone was put into a geriatric ward. There was another case of a child, aged twelve, thrown into a swimming pool to see if he sank. We are speaking here of the most fundamental of civil rights. One of the curious notions some of us with M.E. share is the desire to have MS rather then M.E. This is because civil rights for MS sufferers are slightly higher – not a great deal higher, but higher nonetheless.

With M.E. there is a special and insidious and unpleasant deprivation of rights. It's more like institutionalized apartheid in that one isn't given a chance. When you are a victim of such an illness, you are not in a position either to identify what your rights are or even to hope to campaign for them, because you're ill. If you are told you have no rights because the implication is that you are a liar and a cheat, it's very difficult to fight back. I think it is something that is specific to M.E., and I think the reason that I am refusing to let the subject go and refusing to miss the opportunity of voicing this is because M.E. can suppress your communication skills, and therefore the number of people who can actually speak out with passion are few. We overwork about five doctors who either have M.E., or by virtue of having spent thirty years working on the subject, genuinely understand the condition. There are few 'on the road to Damascus' conversions but I remember the northern consultant who had a reputation for saying M.E. doesn't exist and that it's a load of rubbish – until he developed it. He's now a speaker on the subject, and clearly a very important spokesman, but we are still not hearing from as many people in society as we should. Why is it that M.E. doesn't have more people fighting on its behalf, more Mums, more Dads, more brothers, more sisters as well as more MPs, more actors, more theatre directors? There is so much confusion in the family, amongst friends and employers. There are few voices. I view Clare Francis as a role model, an articulate, well-informed, passionate person – but there are very few Clare Francises.

I may appear to be quite open about almost anything but I'm still coy concerning certain symptoms. I've lived with permanent diarrhoea, for instance, which is fairly antisocial. Sometimes I'm incontinent, or my brain doesn't work. Sometimes I can't read or write. We're not inclined to speak publicly about these problems. Most people with M.E. don't want to use wheelchairs or sticks or the equivalent of guide dogs, or to be seen as requiring support. The public has a strong misconception about M.E. and I suppose as an ex-playwright, I really am fascinated by this. It's taken me several years to get round to the simple formula that M.E. is first cousin to MS. This covers a wide range of suffering, from people who can live with it quite easily and people who are very seriously impaired, but we've a basis for understanding and conversation. What people want is something concrete that enables them to say it's like cancer, it can be terminal. The first thing I say when I'm on the radio, is that the M.E. sufferers who are not speaking on this programme are those in bed, who are deprived of the power of speech, who can't get themselves dressed, and it's our business tell you that they're there.

I think the most difficult thing about rights is to work out the most appropriate form of communicating with the people with whom you have got problems. If you believe that your problems stem from government legislation, from doctors, from the media, then you have to employ different tactics, different language, different timescales, different methods to get across a convincing argument. While we have to admire Clare Francis and her organization and the organization that I was identified with as vice chair, they have not had the staff or the resources or the knowledge for satisfactory lobbying. On the other hand, in the last two years the disability movement has made real progress towards legislation because it's really drawing on the skills of its members, and when it won a lobby outside the House of Commons it was extremely effective. It may all be desperately frustrating but if that's the reality of life, then we have got to find ways of working with those realities.

I think the key to survival is to manage your illness. This is not only the most practical thing you can do, it also puts you in control, which is what makes it positive. If you can manage it, if you can be the boss, then you can live with M.E. and still have a full life, even though there are hours, days, months and even years when it gets the upper hand. I've just come through a month of being largely confined to bed. Although that's a very negative experience, I know that by accepting being in bed, by being in control of my life, then I'm in control of the M.E. and that's what managing is about. It means being practical and realistic enough to recognize the extent of the M.E., the severity of the M.E. and what you might at first call the limitations imposed by it. In a sense M.E. need not be any more inhibiting than other things that we've had to come to terms with. But if you try to pretend, which was my experience initially, and tell people that you are super-heroic, believe you can conquer it by refusing to admit that it exists, or just walk further than you can actually safely walk, you will be disabling yourself as surely as stepping out would disable a wheelchair user.

It sounds very easy and very obvious to be in control of your life but if it means admitting that you can't do things, it's crucial that you don't see that as giving in but as taking control. The severity of M.E. varies with each person, it varies from hour to hour, so it's not an easy thing to come to terms with. Some of the biggest M.E. achievers are those who have it quite severely and who, if they go to some terribly important M.E. meeting or conference and find themselves having a bad attack, will say so and go and lie down for two hours. Think about it in a different way like, for example, if you have a broken leg. Supposing you believed that putting your leg in plaster and resting it and using crutches was giving in, and you insisted on playing football instead, clearly you'd damage your leg for life and you'd have no future as a footballer. You wouldn't dream of doing this and in many ways we are talking about something that ought to be as simple a concept to grasp.

What will give you problems is not accepting M.E., and trying to fight it. The two times I've been hospitalized in an emergency, and the times that I've had major relapses which have put me in bed, reduced all my faculties, made me feel fairly useless for weeks, even months at a time, they have nearly always followed bad planning of my life when I tried to do too much, or got too excited. M.E. is related to adrenalin and the hardest thing for some people is to spot when they are actually becoming ill. Some are lucky and just get more tired and can't speak, but for some of us, we're like hyperactive children. We go over the top into false energy and it ends in tears before the night's out.

Memory loss seems to be a significant component for a lot of people who have M.E. What can be very severe in some cases is short-term memory loss. I have a much older aunt who's recently developed quite severe Alzheimer's. When she was still socially active, we were at the same stage of short-term memory loss, and we sat on a garden wall in the sunshine at my parents' house one day giggling for two hours like small kids (she being about seventy and I about fifty) because we could share and understand the absurdity of, for example, confusing cat with butter or ink with orange juice.

I've said that you have to live within and with the limitations that M.E. imposes on you. As a former marathon runner, I have to accept that using a power wheelchair and a stairlift to get me up the stairs leaves me with more energy to contribute to a social conversation or trying to change the world. I hear a lot of experts on M.E., even some of those with M.E., saying how crucial it is that we take small amounts of exercise. They even advise taking a walk every afternoon, going for a swim or walking the dog. In my experience, this level of exercise would force me to bed all year round with no capacities whatsoever. I think many who have a milder form of M.E. have not quite understood the very real limitations of some M.E. sufferers and that disabled people who have other medical conditions or medical impairments lead totally useful, lengthy and active lives without taking exercise.

What I think is misunderstood by a lot of people who don't have M.E. is that M.E. is such a variable condition. Those of us who have it occasionally get days of remission, days when you feel better, and your first impulse is to do everything to maximum effect. After several years of using a wheelchair, I once woke up feeling so good that I went straight out, got on a bicycle, rode two miles on it and then found myself confined to bed for three months. And yet the moment I felt better my natural desire was to take exercise. Two or three particularly wise doctors on M.E. say that when you are feeling good or better relative to your normal condition, you should sit down and make a really carefully thought out decision about what you want to do with your improved health. Like someone who on their first day of a holiday, asks themselves, do I want to walk in the garden and pick flowers, go to the cinema, iron a shirt, spend some time with my granddaughter, or go and see a play? Make very positive decisions, so that you don't accidentally use up that good time and then afterwards say 'I wish, if only...'

# Darren Guymer

Darren Guymer is twenty-five years old, single and has no children. He used to be a banker but has been unemployed since August 1988. His M.E. began in August 1987 while he was on holiday in Spain. His condition is relatively stable at present but was aggravated by viral meningitis contracted in June 1992. Although Darren uses a wheelchair, he is forced to spend most of his time in bed. He lives in Lowestoft with his parents.

My M.E. started in August 1987. I was on holiday in Spain with five mates, in Benidorm. Three of us fell ill there, just sore throat and diarrhoea and so on but that's not unusual when you travel abroad. The other two got better, no problem, but I travelled home aware that something wasn't quite right. I thought I'd just caught something, probably because of staying out too late, drinking a bit too much. But since then I've been ill.

It took a while for the full syndrome to become established. I had a week off work when I came home, and just thought that I had a foreign flu or whatever, but I was aware that it was a bit more than that. I felt very ill and exhausted. My brain didn't seem to work properly and my legs felt very heavy. After I returned to work, I managed for a few months but I was definitely under par. I had a constant sore throat, heavy muscles, and everything was an extreme effort. Over time it got worse particularly while playing sport. I was once a very active person, working hard during the day as well as studying in the evenings. I also played a lot of sport – squash, tennis, a bit of football. After physical exercise I felt terrible, and within weeks I was going back and forth to the doctor. He did a few tests and said I had a viral infection but that it would go away. As time progressed I was aware that it wasn't going away. I had a lot of pain in my muscles and an overwhelming sense of leaden muscle fatigue. This was much worse even on limited exercise, such as walking a hundred yards, whereas previously I could have walked two or three miles to work or played squash for a few hours. A hundred yards was leaving me feeling completely done in, with a lot of pain in the muscles, visible twitching – a sort of rippling under the skin all over the body – and occasionally the muscles would go into spasm. I had a lot of headaches and was having incredible difficulty functioning at a level which would have been quite normal before.

Work was also becoming a problem. I was on the management development programme and so I was pushing myself to work hard. There was a lot to take in but it was becoming increasingly difficult. I had great difficulty concentrating as well as being in physical discomfort and just feeling ill. The best way to describe it is that my brain wouldn't work properly. My memory was poor and I would forget things easily whereas previously I had been pretty sharp. I'd been used to coming home from work, having my tea, maybe a game of squash and then studying for a few hours for the A levels I was doing, but it just wouldn't go in.

Previously I had been able to study, no problem, I enjoyed it. Now my brain wouldn't accept what I was trying to take in. I was also having other physical symptoms. I had a lot of problems with blurred vision, ringing in the ears, and my glands felt painful. I knew something was drastically wrong so I kept going back to the doctor. To be honest this didn't really get me anywhere. I think he became a bit impatient after he'd done the tests. He'd diagnosed a probable virus and thought that it should have gone away by now. As I returned again and again, he suggested I was working too hard and that perhaps it was stress. But it was overwhelmingly physical. I felt as if I had flu all the time, indeed worse than this, there was so much muscle pain I persisted going back to him saying that something was still wrong.

Moving on into early 1988, performance at work was going downhill even faster. I just wasn't coping. I was having odd days off, sometimes two or three days at a time. I would ring up and say I'm ill, I think I've got another virus. Understandably they became concerned at work. By now I had pretty much stopped all sport as well. I'd had to cancel any squash because it seemed to make me feel worse. It was as much as I could do to get work, do the best I could, get home and crash out! I tried to go out in the evenings because I'd had a good social life before, pubs, night-clubs and so on. But I'd go for an hour and have to say 'I'm sorry, I'm going to pack this in, I'm going home.' Again it was clear to me that something was wrong. It wasn't just that I was struggling at work, my social life was going to pot as well.

Everything was gradually getting worse. The doctors still couldn't come up with anything, and by now, the summer of 1988, I'd booked a holiday abroad. I went to the doctor and said I thought that something was still drastically wrong and I'd booked a holiday. He suggested that a couple of stress-free weeks would probably do the trick. So I went to Magaluf, in Majorca with a group of mates. The flight was terrible. I was having a lot of headaches and pressure in the head and this became intolerable during the flight. On the first day I managed to get to the beach but for the next two or three days I was ill in bed. I was horribly ill. The holiday hadn't helped and I got an early flight home. This pretty much marked the turning point in the whole business.

I had been brought up to trust doctors. But when they are persistently telling you there's nothing wrong, it's stress or it's in your mind, you become disheartened. When I was drastically ill on holiday and had to come back, I returned to the doctor demanding better treatment. He thought I was pressurizing him for some sort of diagnosis and came up with the idea that I suffered from severe anxiety fantasy. I wasn't happy about this because the symptoms were overwhelmingly physical. I'm not saying I wasn't affected psychologically, my concentration had lapsed and I was feeling depressed - after all my life was going to pot. With his say-so I paid privately to see a neurologist. After a neurological examination, the neurologist concluded that I was suffering from something called myalgic encephalomyelitis, M.E. He didn't really explain to me what it was but said it would get better in time.

I tried to return to work in the knowledge that I probably did have this M.E. and I persisted for a few weeks, or a month or so. But then I caught another bug. Again this made everything worse, and so late

August 1988 was the last time I went to work. I went home to Felixstowe, to stay with my parents and got to see a local GP. He confirmed that M.E. probably was the correct diagnosis. He was sympathetic and understanding. He clearly believed that there was an illness called M.E., and that I had it. He was prepared to write certificates of sickness. Finally I informed the bank that I wouldn't be returning.

Over the months that followed I deteriorated still further. I hadn't had any specific advice at this point about how best to deal with the illness, whether to fight it, or rest. But I do believe I was still trying to deny that I was ill. I didn't cope well with not being able to work, or study, or have a social life and no sport. I became bitter, I think, which manifested itself in me trying to fight it by still denying that I was ill. I think now in retrospect this was a mistake. Although in severe pain at the time, with twitching and spasming muscles, I would force myself to walk a mile or whatever, when I wasn't really capable of doing ten yards. Despite the pain worsening – severe headaches, vision deteriorating, throat sorer – I persisted. I could physically do it if I compelled myself.

I felt I had got to keep fit, so I bought a bullworker. I used to sit up in my bedroom doing this, which with the state my muscles were in – they were clearly diseased – was the worst thing I could do. This carried on for several months, even though my GP said I should rest. When I had an appointment at the doctor's, which was more than half a mile away, I would try to walk there even if I had the option of a lift. Even though I wasn't really capable of it, I didn't want to believe that at nineteen I couldn't walk half a mile to the doctor's and back, and so I forced myself to keep going.

Physically I carried on and deteriorated still further. By 1990 I was still ill. Some days I was not capable of walking at all. I might lie on the settee most of one day and feel a bit better the next. Right that's it, I'd go and walk a mile or two. I wanted, obviously, and willed myself, to be better, and I thought the way to do it was to fight and beat it, to be determined. I think in retrospect that this was very foolish, and I suppose I must be honest and say that because I was deteriorating, I wasn't getting any better. I wasn't working. I didn't have a social life and I'd moved away from most of my friends.

The symptoms were still just as severe as ever and I reached the point of considering suicide. I wasn't getting better, but efforts to beat it and fight it were counter-productive. I seriously felt that life wasn't worth living. On the days when I felt slightly better I was quite happy. But the fact that my body wasn't working frustrated me more than anything. I suppose I was a little frightened too. The doctor tried antidepressants but unfortunately they had very bad side effects. I ended up in casualty twice as a result, which apparently isn't uncommon with M.E.

One of the antidepressants caused water retention. I had had problems with my bladder anyway, and still do to this day, but obviously the antidepressants exacerbated the problem. I couldn't urinate and so had to have a catheter. This happened twice. Another time my neck went right into spasm and my chin was pushed down against my chest. Again I had to go into casualty and have an injection which relaxed the muscles; so antidepressants didn't really work.

At this time, probably early 1991, I saw a local consultant who was interested in M.E. He reappraised me and said, 'Look, you've been going about this completely the wrong way. The most important thing with this disease is rest. The muscles are affected badly, and because the hallmark of the disease is muscle fatigue, pain and twitchings on exercise, you need to rest. Don't force yourself to do things. A little exercise around the house and in the garden will be fine.' Over time I did learn to rest and this I think was another turning point. I found it very hard. I won't say I did as strictly as I had been advised. Still, if I'd been resting a bit in the day, I would think to myself, well I must be able to do something, go out, go for a walk, or go out for the evening.

Although probably I didn't do it that well, I did now realize that rest was important and did actually arrest the deterioration. Unfortunately, at least in terms of the muscles, it didn't lead to any improvement: I still had severe and constant pain and muscle fatigue, particularly in the legs, though rest did stop it from getting much worse. The other symptoms, which I'll term the neurological ones – blurred vision, tinnitus, bad headaches, poor concentration and slurred speech – did improve with rest, but the pains didn't.

Over time I levelled out a bit more and the decline was certainly arrested, though I was still unsure of how long I was going to be ill. The specialist told me it would be a while before I could expect signs of any real improvement, so I enrolled for a college course to do an A level. I'd already done an A level part-time while working at the bank as well as taking the banking exams. I thought this would get me back into the swing of things, so I applied to university and was accepted. This entailed three to four hours a day, three days a week at a local college, which I managed for three or four months, perhaps a bit longer. I did pretty well in the essays and so on, but again I think I was pushing it and my condition deteriorated. This was very frustrating, but clearly I had to wind down. I levelled out a bit and decided to try to become more independent. I managed to get a flat. I needed help obviously with some of the physical tasks but I did manage to live by myself for a while. Unfortunately, and this became characteristic, I'd catch another virus and have to return home for a few months with a relapse and have to relinquish the flat. I had three or four flats over the space of a year or two.

This brings me roughly up to the middle of 1992. I was able to live independently, which was very important to me, but I wasn't really making much progress. I wasn't working nor did I have much of a social life. I could perhaps go out once every three months but would pay for it dearly. Even so I had some quality of life. Then in June, I went down very badly with what I thought was another bug – severe headaches, neck pain, stiffness, etc. All the M.E. symptoms were a bit worse but I also had this eye pain and high temperature. After a few days I went into hospital, had a lumbar puncture and eventually was diagnosed as having viral meningitis. This caused an enormous relapse for almost a year. I couldn't stand any light through the curtains, couldn't lift my head very much – the most I could do was to get to the loo and back. I had been pretty ill anyway but with meningitis on top, it felt fairly catastrophic.

I've improved a little since then – most days I can read a bit, I can bear the light, I can get downstairs on very good days and can cope with trips out in the chair – I'm still confined to bed most of the time. The muscle pains and all the M.E. symptoms are just as severe as ever, no worse, no better. I have headaches constantly. Some days I'm feeling worse than others, particularly when I'm reduced to being totally immobile. This more or less brings me up to the present day.

My current main symptom is severe constant muscle fatigue, a leaden acid burning in the muscles, quite different from anything I've ever experienced when well. I used to play squash for three to four hours a time and my muscles had not the slightest feeling of tiredness. Muscle fatigue is now all over the body, but worst in the legs and thighs. There's a severe pain and tenderness not really relieved by painkillers, and a twitching in the muscles. I can feel it sometimes and you can see it rippling under the skin. Occasionally the muscles actually go into spasm. Since the meningitis, I've had constant pain behind the eyes, neck pain and stiffness. These are the consistent symptoms, varying in some degree, but always there. Others which come and go are the blurred vision, tinnitus, pain and problems urinating, sore throats, and painful glands. My bowels have also been affected at times. Occasionally I have poor concentration and memory difficulties but I'm more affected physically than mentally. My speech will be affected if I have a bad day. Sometimes I have trouble even stringing sentences together, although that's relatively rare. Also since the meningitis I've had quite bad nightmares.

In general I would say I'm quite a bubbly person, an optimistic, positive person. I have to say, though, that M.E. has been a negative experience in my life. I was quite an ambitious person and hoped to get on and study and so on, but that option seems to have been taken away from me. But despite the disability, I would say I am still quite positive and bubbly, still optimistic and still fairly ambitious. But however much I try to achieve things, the severity of the M.E. disease process is such that those things are out of my reach at present, so I've had to temper my ambitions a bit.

Overall, my life experience as a result of M.E. has been negative because I do feel I've missed a lot, and the things that were important to me have been thwarted. I don't have relationships, for instance, which was something I enjoyed. There have been some good aspects. I think I was reasonably tolerant anyway and understanding of other people's problems, but clearly I am more so now. I can empathize greatly with other people's problems, not just health problems, but people whose lives haven't turned out the way they'd hoped, and who've had a rough ride. I definitely value the small things that I can do, be it making a cake, seeing pigeons in the park from my wheelchair, writing a letter, or even reading a few chapters of a book. The few things I can do I really enjoy and I appreciate them even though they are things that before I would have totally taken for granted. Clearly, in time, when hopefully I get better, I am really going to appreciate life more than I ever would have done. I think previously I took my health for granted, and now obviously I don't, so it has been positive in that sense.

I would say that I feel cautious when it comes to thinking about my chances of getting better. For the first three or four years I really was utterly convinced that I would be perfectly healthy in a short space of time, and I used to make plans with a view to that. Of course when that didn't happen, I would come down like a ton of bricks, so I suppose I'm now cautiously optimistic. I have to be realistic about it, I've had it seven years, and I'm not any better. In fact in some ways I'm worse, so it's not going to just go away tomorrow. But I haven't lost hope. I think if I lost hope I'd be in a bit of trouble, so I try now to deal with what I've got here and now, make the best of what it is, but still be hopeful and dream of the day when things return to 'normal'.

I have discovered that when I am able, reading is an enjoyable and satisfying pastime, whereas probably previously, what with study, work and social life, I didn't. I have a particular interest in the novels of Thomas Hardy. I don't have that many hobbies. If I try and take an interest or force myself to do something it normally backfires and I end up able to do even less than when I started.

I enjoy cooking very much, like a standard curry, a chilli con carne, or something like that. I like trying out new recipes, cakes, puddings. I'll try my hand at anything really, provided I've got someone to experiment on and who's prepared to risk food poisoning!

My nephew and niece have been born since I've been unwell and I suppose if I'd been fit and well and working, I wouldn't have seen anything like as much of them as I do. It's been a joy and pleasure to see them growing up. I'm very fond of them, and that's been a really positive experience.

I suppose the most unexpected aspect of this debilitating experience has been my ability to cope. I have been surprised also by my family's ability to cope with the unprecedented strain on them. If you'd have said to me seven years ago this is what's ahead for you, I think I probably would have said I won't be able to take it. But, although life is difficult, it's painful, a struggle and I get frustrated, I have coped. I'm here to tell the tale seven years on. The negative side of the unexpected is that people don't accept how I am as it is, neither the medical profession nor the general public. Perhaps this is peculiar to M.E., but I often feel I'm having to justify how I am, excuse it almost, as people don't seem to accept that I'm this ill, that I have this much pain.

I am surprised by this lack of understanding. I find it difficult to believe that anybody could think – and a lot do – that a person of my age would choose to miss out on the things I've missed out on, the things I want to do, the things that other people take for granted. It's not as if I had any choice in the matter. I find it hard to take comments such as, 'Well, it must be nice to lay in bed all day,' or 'It's easy to become dependent on others.' When I hear comments like these, I bite my tongue. Then I just try to explain rationally and logically that that isn't the way it is and that if I could possibly do more, I'd be doing it. The pleasure I get on a day that I can wash up is nobody's business, but people still say that I'm escaping the responsibilities of life, housework, having to get my own meals. I find it hard to believe that they can't see that those responsibilities which I'm supposedly avoiding are actually privileges.

There have been amusing incidents also. I suppose my neck going into a spasm with the antidepressants in its way was funny. I was in town and my neck started to twitch a little and my chin was pushing down. As I was walking along the street I couldn't hold my chin up so I kept knocking into people, sort of head-butting people. I'm sure they thought I was either drunk or I don't know quite what, but I just found it enormously funny at the time. I couldn't really see where I was going and I was head-butting people left, right and centre! I had to come home in the car, my mother drove me. I had a lie down and thought it was a little bit better but as I stood up my chin went down again. I tried to make myself a cup of tea and managed to put the kettle and the teapot on the floor and smashed the mug. Then I decided that it was time to call the doctor.

Another time, again concerning odd reactions to the drugs, was about three years ago when I had two fillings at the dentist. I sat in the chair and was given an anaesthetic. I've got quite a wide jaw bone so they had to give me a large dose and I felt quite relaxed. When it was over, I could hardly put one foot in front of the other. I felt completely off my head, drunk if you like but very light-headed. I stumbled out of the place, giggling, I couldn't stop laughing. The receptionist asked me to pay, and when I went into my pocket to get the money out, I threw it on the floor which I thought was enormously funny. I was high, I suppose, and again my Mum gave me a lift home. I was talking nonsense in the car, my mouth all swollen so I was slurring the words, and she was creasing up; she had to stop the car three times she was laughing so much.

Once when I was at my parents', I was looking after the dog while they were away. My memory is not at its best and I found out afterwards that I'd inadvertently fed the dog three times in the same day. I became aware of it in the evening because he was lying on his back with his four legs in the air, his stomach about three times the size of normal. I got in a bit of a muddle there.

Just existing and coping with day-to-day problems is an achievement. My achievements tend to be intangible, such as keeping my sense of humour. I have some great laughs and I keep an interest in the outside world that goes by past my window. It's interesting that previously when I was well, I got ten O levels, six grade As, and when I did an A level in the evenings over a period of five months, which meant studying all hours of the night, I got a grade A. Things like this are achievements, but in my opinion it takes more determination, commitment, will-power and strength to cope with just two weeks of being in the position I am now in compared with all those previous achievements put together.

Early on I did try to go swimming which badly backfired. I managed two or three times, but eventually had to give up. There have been other things that I have tried and wanted to do. But obviously I'm restricted and I haven't yet really come to terms with this. Often I attempt to mobilize myself and make almost heroic attempts to get myself going on better days. Inevitably it seems I fall short. If I read two chapters of a book yesterday, I'd want to read two chapters today, but the headache or the vision would be so bad that I couldn't take the sentences in. There are definite failures imposed by the severity of my M.E.

I've tried desperately to hang on to a normal life and have tried to sustain as much of the fullness of life that I had before. I can't think that there's anything I haven't done – although sport is another matter. Initially I tried to motivate myself but now it is completely out of the question. We are talking about a walk of twenty yards being equivalent to struggling up a mountain.

Before the meningitis, I did go to football matches at Norwich, that is before I was as bad as this. I was determined that I would go to see a game. I've got a mate who funnily enough was an Ipswich supporter, but he didn't mind going to Norwich. I used the wheelchair and went just that once but paid severely for it. I am determined that I will get back to Carrow Road where Norwich play - the temple - and I'm sure I will. You have to be determined. Even now I could say, right I'm going to spend one evening in the pub with a friend, but I'd then be capable of doing so much less for weeks afterwards. Experience has taught me that it's a balancing act between doing the small things and being able to do them on a consistent basis. Attempting something monumental and then not even being capable of the most minimal things afterwards is a constant trial and error thing. I'm still learning.

Since I first became ill at eighteen/nineteen, I've not really had any relationships, not even so much as a date. Obviously being stuck in here, I miss not only having relationships but female company of my own age. It's also been difficult to make new friends here because of not being able to get out. I passed my driving test when I was 17 and did have a car. I used to enjoy driving very much, it gave me a lot of independence. I've always valued my independence. I do feel a great sense of loss, because obviously I have the same physical and emotional desires and needs as anybody of my age. When these aren't met I get lonely and frustrated. I haven't lost hope but clearly it's difficult.

I have one sister who's four years older than me and she lives quite nearby. She has a little boy and girl. I see something of them. I'm very close to my sister and have had a lot of support from her. She's a social worker so she is able to help me apply for State benefits, fill in forms, get a wheelchair and a disabled badge. She was also a great help when I applied for housing benefit.

I've never had a great desire to have children, so the fact that I may not be able to have them doesn't worry me too much. But because I was only nineteen when the M.E. started, I haven't really thought it through. Maybe long term I probably would have thought it was a possibility, but I don't as yet feel a sense of loss or any desire or frustration that I can't have them. In time, of course, I may feel differently, time will tell. At present I enjoy seeing my friends'and sister's children, but they can be very tiring.

I've been quite fortunate on the whole with my friends. Of a big circle of friends quite a lot of them have kept in contact to this day, seven years on. Some have fallen by the wayside, so to speak, but quite a few keep in regular contact, phone calls and visits from time to time. One friend in particular, Steve, has been absolutely brilliant. He phones every week whether I'm capable of speaking on the phone or not, so for months he might only speak to my Mum but this doesn't deter him. He'll visit whenever I am up to it, irrespective of what's going on in his life. He makes the time and that's been great, though often it's a case of him just coming round here and sitting with me or whatever.

As far as employment is concerned I'm still hopeful and optimistic that in time I will be able to work either part-time or full-time. Although given how I am now, I don't know whether this is a realistic prospect. Hopefully, if my health allows, I'd like to go back to university, possibly to study something like Politics, Philosophy, and Economics.

On the whole my experience of the medical profession has been mixed. Some doctors and consultants are interested in M.E. and believe it's a genuine neurological condition and want to learn about it. I think that's important. I've also met some at the other extreme, and have faced outright hostility, ridicule, and total disbelief. There are also those doctors who sit in the middle and sort of misunderstand what it is.

When I realized that conventional medicine didn't have an awful lot to offer I did seek the answer in alternative therapy. I spent an awful lot of money and tried anything that I could think of: homeopathy, royal jelly, faith healing, spiritual healing, Efamol Marine, oil of evening primrose, various special diets, an anti-candida diet, i.e. eliminating sugar and yeast, pro-biotics (they use a substance which supposedly puts back the good bacteria into the gut), vitamins and mineral supplements, and a new device which alters brain-wave patterns and corrects those that are apparently incorrect (it's a little disc that you hold around your neck which was supposed to correct brain waves).

But I can't say that any of these alternative treatments have been of any real help. M.E. is an up-and-down thing anyway so it's difficult to assess whether something has or hasn't helped. But for sure nothing has been dramatic and I haven't felt the benefit, not to mention my bank balance. Initially, in the first year or two that I was ill, I believed there had to be an answer or magical cure and every time I heard of something, I'd rush into it like a headless chicken. When it didn't work you'd come down quite hard particularly when you've hoped that it would be a miracle cure. I'm more cautious now, although it has to be said that if there is something that offers the slightest chance I do tend to have a go.

The only thing that I'm trying at the moment is a TeNS machine which is also I believe used conventionally by the NHS, by physios and in pain-relief clinics and so on. It's not even promising to improve anything, but it's to help with the severity of the pain. I still take Efamol Marine which is fish oil, plus oil of evening primrose and Vitamin E. I've taken them on and off for over three or four years but I haven't noticed any difference. I'm always hopeful that something helpful will materialize either conventionally or in alternative treatment.

My life is more difficult than it was before. I cope on a day-to-day, week-to-week basis. I think my philosophy now is just to take each day as it comes and not to think too much about the next one. This is difficult at times but generally I manage it. When I was still in a flat the home-helps were invaluable because they took care of the physical housework which I was unable to do. They did shopping and so on for me. I think probably the understanding of the GP and consultant too has given immeasurable support in the face of so much hostility.

Once I went to a psychologist in the belief that perhaps it would be helpful; it wasn't. I'm sure this person was doing their best and had good intentions, but the attitude was rather dismissively to advise me to get on with life and compel myself to do things. As I explained earlier, this kind of misjudgment always proved counter-productive.

Emotionally, I would say I've been fairly up and down. There have been moments of utter desperation. There's been a lot of frustration as I've had to adjust to what I was losing and what I could no longer do and how life was changing. This was on top of the physical pain and suffering. But once I'd found a sympathetic and understanding consultant and GP, and I'd learnt a bit more about M.E., I had to accept my condition. I have come to terms with it over time since then.

It's been very difficult for my parents. To begin with, it was very difficult to return home and reestablish a relationship with my parents. It was stressful for me and for them. One's basic expectation is that by the early twenties you are independent of your family, but I can't be. I'm at home now, and it is difficult. We've all had to adjust. I have to live by the way they live, for example, I can't live my own lifestyle. I know I would have had a different kind of life to what I have here with my parents. We're on top of one another, all being in the same house, which compromises their lifestyle as well. I mainly occupy one room, so I'm restricted anyway, but because I need a certain amount of care they have to take account of that, so their lives have changed dramatically too. Although they don't show it, I'm sure there's an element of, if not resentment, certainly frustration. They are coping much better now than they did initially. At the start it was an unexpected thing to see their son not being able to fulfil the things he wanted to do and what they wanted. I was in a lot of pain and unhappy, which was very hard for them. I would guess, like me, their way of coping is to try not to think too much of the things that I can't do, and that other people of my age do, but to enjoy the things I can do. Like when I have a slightly better day I can get downstairs or when I can be taken to a park. We appreciate and get as much out of this as we can.

On the whole my parents think I've coped reasonably well. I think it surprised them as much as it has me that I can cope with this lifestyle because of the type of person they knew me to be. At the start they probably thought as I do that I didn't cope very well but, in retrospect, because I became frustrated and wouldn't give in, I tried to fight it. I was expending all my energy on fighting, getting frustrated and feeling bitter, and I think it was understandable perhaps that none of us coped well to start with. But over time we've coped better because we've had to.

At present I get invalidity benefit, which helps. I also get a mobility allowance as I'm not able to walk very far, and a disability living allowance, which is a care allowance. This is because to some extent I'm dependent on others for some of the bodily functions and so on. I have had to battle quite hard for these benefits at times, because of the condition fluctuating so much. When, occasionally, I could walk quite a distance, I was refused the mobility allowance twice. I got accepted on appeal eventually, but as with the other allowances, it has been a battle. You have to chase things up, make phone calls, write letters, fill in a tumult of forms and so on. I've been fortunate and had people who have helped me with endless form-filling that I wouldn't have been able to do on my own. I imagine that it's horrendous for people who haven't got the support of family or friends. Occasionally you're reassessed for these benefits which can mean seeing other doctors. This has been problematic at times because they have either not understood or believed in the illness M.E.

My mother had to give up work to look after me following the meningitis, so the financial assets I receive are our sole income. The invalidity benefit is £68 a week, the mobility allowance £30, and the care allowance is £20.

In general, though, I'd like to see changes in the application for benefits and form filling. While I appreciate the need to ascertain that you are a genuine candidate, I do think some of the form-filling could be reduced. Often, after a few months I have to reapply and fill in all the same forms again for a benefit I am already receiving. This is an unnecessary strain that could, and ought, to be avoided.

The discrimination that I experience is apparent in that some people simply don't see me as genuinely disabled. When you say you've got M.E. you often aren't believed or it's interpreted as a euphemism for lazy or apathetic or whatever. Research, and better education would, I believe, encourage a more tolerant view. In general, the preconception of M.E. is that it is not a genuine physical illness but malingering, total nonsense. It's difficult to support what is backed simply by anecdotal evidence. I believe research is being undertaken to show that there are organic abnormalities and that steps have been taken to prove that this is a genuine organic disease. Another problem lies in the fact that M.E. can be over-diagnosed. If you look at the papers written by M.E. experts, it is a specific diagnosis. But it's become a bit of a dustbin diagnosis. Here I think is the danger. A lot of people have unexplained health problems, so often doctors diagnose M.E. This, I believe, can prejudice research and probably fuels some of the disbelief and misconceptions about M.E.

Dr Ramsay, a consultant at the Royal Free Hospital in the mid-1950s, at the time when nearly 300 members of staff and patients fell ill with what would seem to have been M.E., dedicated the rest of his life to the illness. Shortly before his death a few years ago, his main concern was that M.E. was not differentiated and distinguished from other post-viral states. Feeling rough after a virus can last for months, even a year or two with things like hepatitis. But this is quite different from M.E. Other chronic fatigue states or tired-all-the-time syndrome are different again. Dr Ramsey was concerned that M.E. wasn't being identified as a unique disease in its own right. I'm not saying the other conditions aren't worthy of being understood and helped, but there is confusion. The change I'd like to see is the clarification of M.E. made central to the research of what distinguishes it from other conditions.

People still confuse M.E. with 'yuppie flu'. It's a legacy of the tabloid press, I think, and it's done a great deal of harm. If you look at the statistics, people who have M.E. aren't necessarily yuppies at all. I hope in time the term 'yuppie flu' will become obsolete.

I think it will all become clearer when the medical profession is better educated and able to diagnose exactly what M.E. is. Education of the general public through the media would also help. Often when illnesses first emerge in the public eye, there's a lot of misunderstanding and scepticism. Legionnaire's disease and multiple sclerosis, for example, were dismissed in the early stages of their materialization. Even AIDS: I saw a programme recently in which people with HIV or AIDS were dismissed as malingerers with a sort of 'lifestyle' condition.

These drastic misconceptions are due, I think, to the failure of the medical profession and the media to inform the general public. Probably the medical profession panics when something comes along that is mysterious and incurable. I remember somebody saying to me once, 'Don't catch anything unless it's in the medical textbooks.' I appreciate that doctors have an incredible amount to learn about, and that there's a lot they only touch on in medical school, but what about showing a little more humanity, flexibility and understanding? A little open-mindedness wouldn't go amiss.

My advice to someone with M.E. would be to rest – or to listen to your body. Doctors who have had decades of experience with M.E. advise rest, complete rest. Then gradually increase what you do but still listen to your body. It's important to try and live within the limitations the disease imposes and not to keep trying to push beyond them, which is what I did. I think almost without exception those who make good improvements and indeed recover from M.E., are those who've rested at the start and have been able very gradually to rehabilitate themselves within the limits the disease imposes. If you live within those limits, evidence shows that those limitations should decrease and you have a better chance of recovering. Again, without exception, it seems to me that those who are severely disabled long-term by M.E. are those who didn't receive or heed that advice. They pay the price in terms of long-term disability. On the whole it's sensible to listen to your body and to try to gradually increase what you do within the limitations of the illness.

What you shouldn't do is try to beat it. It's difficult early on and quite frightening to accept the limitations, but you are ill and should not deny it because in my experience this doesn't work. You also need to see a doctor who is understanding and who is going to assess you to see if M.E. is genuinely what you have. This is not as easy as it sounds, because of the continuing misunderstandings. You should conserve energy where you can, get as much help as you can, conserve energy rather than fight in the way that I did.

I also think that even though I spent a lot of money on alternative help that didn't work, I wouldn't say it was money wasted. It was a process I had to go through in search of answers. I'm sure that other newly diagnosed people, irrespective of what I or anyone else says, would want to find out for themselves. But my advice would be to be a little bit cautious. I'm sure there are plenty of genuine people in the alternative field but, regrettably, it is open season for the charlatans. Because M.E. isn't understood, sufferers are suggestible targets for experimenting practitioners.

Patience is of key importance. You've got to realize that anything is going to take time, whether it's an improvement or even an alternative therapy. An answer tomorrow is unrealistic. Obviously I hope I'm going to improve over time and that my quality of life improves and I will become less ill and more active. Whether that will happen or not remains to be seen. I would say I was cautiously optimistic, which ties in with my other hopes – regaining independence, forming relationships and having girlfriends, even work, study and travel. All these things I haven't lost hope of achieving. But I have had temporarily to suspend them because it's futile to suppose that next year or next month I will be able to do them.

To a point, I'm trying to live in the present with what I have got. But I'm still hopeful of returning to a comparatively normal life. It seems unlikely that this will come through my own body healing as I've been ill for such a long time and been so very disabled. The pain in the muscles has not changed after seven years, so expecting it to stop is, I suppose, unreasonable. I hope for medical intervention and research, and in the immediate future I guess I hope I can just carry on coping and adjusting and living the best I can with M.E.

# Luke Merchant

Luke is nine years old and was diagnosed as having M.E. in March 1993 although his parents suspect he has had it for longer than that - possibly since he was four years old. He was born with a pancreas problem which, although uncured, no longer creates difficulties for him.

He uses a wheelchair when he goes out of the house to help him conserve his energy. He has a home tutor for 5 hours and 15 minutes a week. He has a sister called Hannah who is three, and a foster brother, Daniel, who is sixteen. He lives in Essex.

My name is Luke and I got M.E. sixteen months ago. We went on an activity holiday and when I got home I was exhausted. Mummy and Daddy came home exhausted too but they got over it and I didn't. My mum took me to the doctor who said that I had M.E. I had acupuncture which was a bit frightening; they said they were going to put some needles in my back and I'd never heard of an acupuncturist. Some people have needles stuck in their head. I didn't want to have this done and I don't want to go again but I don't know if I will or not.

When I was ill it hurt everywhere. I started off seeing double, so that I would see two chairs instead of one, for example, and I would try and sit on the wrong one and fall on the floor. The double vision lasted about two months. I also got headaches which felt like electric shocks. I still get these occasionally. My arms hurt sometimes and my heart starts going very fast, which is a bit scary. I have pins and needles in my hands and sometimes in just one finger. It's not easy to explain these things and I don't think my friends really understand it, because I don't really. They know I get lots of aches and pains and that there are things I would like to do but can't. I'd really like to be able to ride a bike. Somebody broke my bike but when I get better some people are going to give me a new one. I'll ride it in the park. I don't like football much, but I like swimming. I don't do it now but I used to do it every Monday at school. I've only done my grade one, you have to make yourself sink under water and see how long you can stay under. You need to stay under for 10 seconds. It is not frightening, because I can swim under water.

There are other things I'd like to do but can't. I'd like to go to Portugal. We were going to go but then I didn't really want to because I didn't think I could handle it. I didn't think I was ready but now I do want to go. We went to EuroDisney two years ago. We were staying in France and we went there for the day. I went on loads and loads of rides. We went in a maze that was made of hedges, we saw the Queen of Hearts and we saw Mickey Mouse and Minnie Mouse, Donald Duck, Jiminey Cricket and Cinderella's castle. At night-time all of the floats were lit up in the night and you could see them.

I used to do horse-riding but I don't anymore because of not being well. I could do massive jumps. I fell off loads of times because the horse bucked me off. I like computers; things like Game Boy and I've got a Sega Master System as well. I really like Super Mario 2 and Sonic. I read some comics but I don't read as much as I used to. I don't think I can concentrate that well. I can only read a page at a time. It's not really a problem for school work but I do need to concentrate for that. A tutor comes to my house so I don't have to go to school. My tutor comes at 9 o'clock.

It's difficult to get up in the morning. Usually I'm really tired and it depends if I've slept well that night. Once, although my tutor was there, I slept until 2 o'clock in the afternoon. I just thought it was about 8 o'clock and I went downstairs and got quite a shock.

My tutor is nice. He understands if I'm tired out or something. He does origami with me and I like writing stories about my favourite friends, Robert and Nicky. I do mathematics, geography, history, science and experiments. Once with origami my tutor made a cup out of paper and we tested to see if it would take water and it did. I'd like to go back to school though because I enjoyed it so much. I'm not saying I'm fed up with Mum, but I'd like to meet other friends.

My wheelchair is helpful. It's easier than walking because I get pains when I walk. My friends don't mind my wheelchair. First of all I had this very slow one and then I got a sports one which is blue. I went into class and all my friends said, 'Wow'. Some people stare at me in my wheelchair, but I don't take any notice. People ask why I'm in a wheelchair and I just say because my legs hurt.

Once I told my friend Josie that I'd got M.E. and he thought it meant a mental illness. He'd never heard of M.E. I tried to explain but it's difficult.

I'm not really worried about falling behind with my school work because I went into school with my old teacher and we'd been doing some work, sums, and I saw that my class had been doing the same things. I was quite pleased with that. It helps being taught one-to-one. I do forget things though. It makes me angry that I can't do things.

I couldn't have bread or milk once. I had to have skimmed milk and all these other things because I've got a bad pancreas. But now I take tablets so I can eat anything.

I get angry about not being able to walk very well because my legs are not very good. I get angry with my sister. I think it's because she's well and I'm not. I don't get angry with Mum....well, I get angry with her sometimes. I don't know why really. I get frustrated.

When I fell ill I felt like I wanted to die. I just wanted to get rid of my M.E. I often feel like I want to die. At Easter I didn't feel very well. I had a lot of pains and a lot of headaches and aches all over and I was tired. I told Mum and Dad I wanted to die and they were upset. I don't know if I really wanted to though. Probably when I die it will be even more painful. I cry a lot because I'm sad when I've got M.E. but I try and hide it from people. I do think my M.E. is going to get better. I can't have it for that long because you can't have it for your whole life, can you? I've got a little bit better. I think my pains have gone down a bit. I'm looking forward to being well. It would make me happier. I can't really remember what it was like when I was well before, it was such a long time ago. When I grow up I want to be a doctor - a GP. I want to be able to make people better.

# Sue Merchant

We believe, looking back, that Luke probably had M.E. when he was four. It was then that we met Dr Franklin who is a paediatric consultant at St John's Hospital in Chelmsford, and he also believes that Luke may well have had it then. Obviously we can't be sure now, as time has passed since, but he prescribed then, when Luke was four, a regimen of vitamins and minerals and said to us that in a year's time Luke would be a lot better. Sure enough, he was a lot better and although he has a pancreas problem we just carried on as if it was OK. Then, during Christmas 1992, we went on an activity holiday; we all came home tired, but Luke just carried on being tired. Even his school began to notice that Luke wasn't Luke. He'd always been a child who liked his sleep but bringing him home from school he'd fall asleep in the car. He'd then come into the house and curl up on the settee and go to sleep. I used to wake him up and he'd just about manage some tea, and then he'd be in bed fast asleep at six o'clock and you'd have to shake him awake the next morning at quarter to eight to get him ready for school.

Between January and March 1993, he had quite a lot of time off school, and in the February half term it was suggested he had another week off hoping that the fortnight might pull him round. Things just got worse, however; the headaches became intolerable, and he became very nauseous. We saw Dr Franklin again in March and I saw him on my own, and by the end of our conversation I knew that Luke had M.E., never having thought about it before.

Dr Franklin interrupted me while we were talking and said could he ask me some questions which I think were designed by one of the Welsh health authorities. It's done on a scoring basis; you have to give so many points for the questions asked and when you add up the score it gives an indication. All the things that he was asking just somehow made me feel that that's what he was going to say was wrong with Luke. In a sense it was a relief, because we knew then what was actually wrong, and so therefore we could start to do something about it. The initial thing to do as far as Dr Franklin could see was to withdraw Luke from school and to give him a regimen of vitamins and minerals again, which is what we started to do.

Luke was eight and three quarters then. He found it quite hard because he loved school, but at the same time he couldn't cope with it. Before that he himself had stopped wanting to go to Cubs, stopped wanting to go horse-riding, both of which he thoroughly enjoyed. He was withdrawing himself from these and other activities because he just couldn't cope with them.

Within our family unit there is my husband and myself, a foster son who is just sixteen, and a little girl who will be three tomorrow. I would say out of all of us the one who has suffered most as a result of Luke's M.E., apart from Luke himself, is Hannah; she was very young and her life became centred around Luke. In fact Hannah wouldn't talk and her health visitor actually thought she'd got learning difficulties because she was so withdrawn. Last September, when we were on holiday in Wales, we decided that we ought to put her into a nursery to give her some time with little children of her own age, and to help stimulate her. Within a month she wasn't only talking words but she was having real conversations with us; she has just blossomed and come into her own.

I was on the fortnight induction course working nights as a care officer for an organization called SESNHA (the South Essex Special Needs Housing Association) when it was discovered that Luke was ill with M.E. It wasn't easy deciding whether to carry on or to stay at home twenty-four hours a day. But I decided, having talked with my husband, that at the end of the day we all had to have a life, and that what we were going to try to maintain was as normal a life as possible. This meant that I would carry on working.

For me the difficulty is trying to split yourself in lots of directions, to make sure that everybody gets a bit of quality time. As a result Mum and Dad sometimes get pushed out. But hopefully, we are strong enough to stand up. In the beginning, when Luke was first told, his little lip dropped. Dr Franklin felt it was better that he told Luke and he explained the problem in as kind a way as possible. As we came home, Luke was incredibly quiet, he didn't want to talk about it. I didn't go into work the next day but stayed at home because I knew that he would break down and cry at some stage. I felt it was right that either Mum or Dad was there for that. He did break down and cry and he got very upset because he then began to realize that there was a reason why he couldn't do the things he wanted to do. We tried to answer his questions as honestly as we could while trying not to create any fears. Initially he coped really well, but at the moment he's fairly disheartened.

There's a lot of frustration which most people with M.E. probably feel – you want to do something and you know you can't. When you're only nine you want to be kicking a ball or out riding your bike like your friends.... When asked what he wants to do most, it's always to ride his mountain bike. That's his goal, and that's quite a choker, because we know he can't. He wouldn't have the strength in his legs. If he hasn't got the strength in his legs to walk around, then how would he have the energy to ride a bike?

No one ever wants to see their child ill and I don't say 'Why Luke?' but I do say 'Why a child?' If there's any sense in this at all, then hopefully we can all be positive and pool our views, our thoughts and any knowledge that we gain together. Then one day, children and adults won't suffer quite as much, because I think that one of the things that people suffer from most with M.E. is ignorance. There is still so much ignorance. We've been very lucky, because we have got a brilliant paediatrician who specializes in M.E., who understands M.E., who is superb with children, and who is always at the end of the phone whenever you want him. For that, we shall always be incredibly grateful.

I don't know how long it will take for Luke to get better. Initially we were told a minimum of five years, but it could be ten, or fifteen. We also understand that there are lots of sufferers that don't ever actually get completely better. Whether that will be Luke, I wouldn't like to say, because I don't think too much towards the future. Somehow you've got to cope with today, and I think that's how you have to look at M.E.: live for today, look to tomorrow, but don't plan too far ahead. I think Luke is very confused and quite frightened because of the uncertainty. A child likes to have structure, and there isn't any real structure. Unfortunately, because of the nature of the beast, and how it affected Luke, he hasn't really wanted to have any other interests which might give his life more structure. I think what we are trying to do is just to give him as much support and love as we can.

People can be prejudiced about M.E. You get odd comments. I heard only this week, 'Oh well, you look at him and you don't think there's much wrong with him,' and my friend's reply to that was, 'You don't know what goes on behind the face.' I think that's very true for M.E. People don't know what goes on behind the face. The wheelchair is, of course, a typical symbol of disability, but the way we tried to look at it was that we wanted to carry on doing as much as we possibly could as a family. Luke couldn't manage walking around, so having the wheelchair enabled him to have some quality life and that in a sense was more important.

At the moment, the thing that my husband and I are struggling with is how Luke has been psychologically. I wonder where we might have gone wrong, but we keep being assured that it's just the way the M.E. is with Luke. But when you look at your child and you see how he has changed so dramatically in personality, you can't help but question whether there's something that you've done wrong. In all honesty I don't think that we have, I just think it's a natural thing to do to question yourself.

I think Andy and I are lucky that we've got the relationship we have. A lot of relationships do break down when people have illnesses, and you have to be very conscious of allowing time for each other. We actually made a very conscious decision at the end of last year that once a month we would go out for a night because we just weren't going out at all. You need to get away from the situation at times. You've got to remember that you're all valued members of the family. Although one person has M.E., the whole family feels like they live it. That's how we perceive it, as does Dr Franklin. We were planning to go to Portugal last year. It was Luke who took the decision that he didn't feel he could cope, so that meant none of us went. We don't get as much out of life as we could because we want to keep the unit tight together. That is the choice that we have made, but other families might decide differently. I think what is important is that there aren't any golden rules. You have to find what suits you as a family the best, and live your lives the best way that you can.

Instead of going to Portugal last year we went to Wales. We would normally just have driven to Wales, but we didn't; we stopped half-way there, and half-way coming back. We hired a cottage in September for a fortnight, but it was then that we actually realized what Luke couldn't do.

Being away from home and from everything that was normal, it all became clear. When we go on holiday we like to do a lot of walking, but it's not so easy to walk with a wheelchair because there are a lot of gates and fences in the way. It was quite funny really, because we got into all sorts of funny situations, wheelchair and all, and made the best of it. I'm glad there wasn't a cine camera following us! Going up little tracks, you walk single file, and at the time the wheelchair wasn't as good as the one he has now, and it kept slipping into ditches. You just take it for granted when you go for a walk that you can get down to a beach or a cove, but life is quite different in a wheelchair. It's a lesson in acquiring a hell of a lot of patience. You take for granted that you've got a healthy child and that your child can do everything they want to do and it's not until they can't that you realize just how awful that is.

We have said that if we hadn't gone on that activity holiday... but then, who knows, it might have come anyway. One of the known factors for the development of M.E. is extreme activity, and it was a very active holiday there: at the grand old age of thirty-four I learnt to ride a bike and we rode for miles and miles. Luke swam and swam, and we had the most wonderful week. If we can put the M.E. out of our minds, it's a holiday we look back on as really great.

We have been really fortunate with Luke's education. We often say that the day Luke's first home tutor was sent to us, a guardian angel was looking down because they could not have sent a kinder man. He has such compassion, he's become a real friend to Luke. He wraps him up in his arms, he tells him he loves him and it's genuine. He's done far more for Luke than was ever necessary. Luke just couldn't cope with school, so Peter has done all sorts of things with him to broaden his interests in other ways. They've made lots of things with origami. Peter will sit with one piece of paper and Luke will sit with the other, and they'll work it through together. He really has been very good and we'll never be able to thank him enough for all his input. Luke does see his friends occasionally, but they want to be doing things nine-year-old boys do, and Luke can't really participate. Boys want to be kicking a ball around, and Luke will go out and try really hard but then he'll pay for it for weeks. Often Luke will make a decision not to do something because he knows that it will have an adverse effect.

Last summer I tried to take him back to horse-riding for a single lesson on his own. I explained to them what the situation was so they were fully aware and they were really good, they accommodated the situation really well. He was on the horse for only half an hour before he looked really ill. I kept thinking was this kindness or was I actually being a bit unkind. He got off the horse and said, 'Mummy, I just can't do it, I'm just so tired.' It took him a good couple of weeks to get over it. You never know how long things are going to go on, you have to try things again from time to time.

The problems that you encounter when you are caring for someone who has M.E. will be different for everyone. Everybody is an individual and everybody's needs are different. There will be similarities, but I think it's very important to remember people are individuals.

We have people who help us. We have a lady who comes in most weeks which means that I can go out and have a couple of hours away. We've had support from people who've had experience of M.E. talking to Luke and trying to help him come to terms with it. From Luke's point of view that's been good, because for him, someone who understands is going to be someone who's had M.E. or who's got it, because as much as we try to understand Luke, it's difficult for us. One lady took Luke out one day and she bumped her car. She said something that you wouldn't normally say to a nine-year-old: 'Oh, never mind Luke, you won't remember because you've got M.E.,' and that was a joke between the two of them! Being able to have a bit of a laugh about it has been good. One of our biggest supports, in all honesty, has been the consultant; I think if you've got a good consultant then you're half-way there. But what we have found useful, another family might not. You have to find your own level, what suits you, and you should grab whatever you can. There is support out there, and I think you don't have to be afraid to ask for it.

Perhaps one of the things that has been most helpful recently is the Specscan. I understand it's only available at the moment at North Middlesex Hospital in London, and Luke actually had a Specscan in September. Although in the consultant's eyes and in ours there wasn't any doubt about M.E., there wasn't any clinical proof, but the Specscan reveals something in black and white. Adults with M.E. still come across with great distrust and disbelief, but with this scan they've then got it in black and white and are not looked on as malingerers. I think that's of great value. The parents of children with M.E. and adults who've got M.E. have got to fight together to get across that there is such a thing as M.E. and that more money needs to be spent on research.

We were advised that we should go for invalidity and attendance allowance. We thought we didn't actually need the money for ourselves, but that if Luke did get it, then we would have put it into some savings' account for him, not knowing how things would be in the future. In fact we were turned down.

I think, over all, we've coped pretty well with our situation, but the last few weeks have been quite difficult because Luke has reached quite a low point. When he feels really down he says he wants to die and when a child of nine is saying that to you, although not necessarily directly, you know what they are actually getting at. It makes me feel absolutely desperate, because it's so sad to think that he feels that's the only way to get rid of it. You just wish it was you instead of him which I think is something that a lot of parents say. We both wish that he could do all the things he wants to do, and we could say to him it will all be over in five years or whatever. But something we've tried to do is be honest with him and if he weren't better he would find it hard to trust our word again. It's important that there is a trust between us.

My husband jokes sometimes about us winning an Oscar for keeping a smile on our faces but when it's a child you've really got to try. If they see you're worried, if they see that you're not coping – you're not helping them. You've got to do the screaming and shouting when they're not around, you've got to let your feelings out.

Luke's memory loss presents problems at times. He gets quite adamant that he hasn't said something or that he hasn't done something. In fact it wasn't until January of this year that he actually remembered that we'd been away the previous Christmas. He'd completely forgotten, and it suddenly came back to him one morning when we were eating breakfast. Without belittling it, you have to try and react light-heartedly, otherwise you'd get terribly depressed.

I think Daniel, our sixteen year old, has handled it all very sensitively and he's actually been very supportive of Luke, I said earlier that Hannah had difficulty in talking but what she quickly picked up on was the names of the tablets Luke was taking. Now she is going around saying, 'Luke's crying again, Luke's sad, Luke's not well, when will Luke be better?' She's only three tomorrow, and when you listen to that, you realize that he is having quite a profound affect on her.

As far as doctors are concerned we've tended to stick mainly with Dr Franklin because there are a lot of medics who still don't understand a great deal about M.E. We did try acupuncture and I think if Luke could have persevered, I honestly think it might have had some effect, but we had to stop it in the summer because he went into hospital. The acupuncturist explained to us that one of the first things you have to do to help someone with M.E. is to get the body warm. When you touch Luke, he's cold, but after he'd had acupuncture for a few weeks, plus the Chinese herbs, his whole body was warm. Now that's not mind over matter it must have done something. Also, when Luke was in hospital he said to me one day, 'You know what, Mummy, my body is all cold again, and it had been warm,' so he'd actually noticed it himself. We gave it a good crack of the whip, but it wasn't for Luke, although I do know that a lot of people with M.E. have been helped greatly by acupuncture.

I hope one day we can all turn round and say that we've gained something from this experience. That sounds a bit back to front in one sense, but hopefully Luke will become a stronger person and it will help him to have an understanding of people. He's always been quite sensitive to other people's needs, but I think and hope that when this is over, the angry feelings he's got at the moment will turn into positive feelings.

The Luke that we live with now isn't the Luke that we knew for the first few years of his life. He was never an angry or upset child, he was a very happy-go-lucky child, and the M.E. has taken that away. We hope that's only temporary.

# Mary Owen

Mary Owen is a grandmother. She has had M.E. since 1987 and her condition varies from day to day, although she feels she is better now than she was during the first two years. She is retired and lives in South London.

The M.E. started in 1987. Whereas with flu which I thought I'd got, you usually recover in a week to ten days, I was just getting worse. I had no energy. I didn't want to eat or do anything. It frustrated me because usually with illnesses I've been able to work through them but with this I couldn't work through at all. I didn't know what was happening to me. I couldn't walk. I had pains in my chest, pains in the muscles of my legs, headaches and I had vertigo. When I stood up everything spun so I thought I'd stay sitting in a chair. Someone who worked in a chemist recommended a tonic that the Jamaicans swear by. I said 'fine, great, I'll give it a go'. I think I had four bottles of the stuff and it seemed to give me a bit more energy. I thought, 'I'm on my way now, so let's get the house cleaned.' I started to do the housework. I cleaned the place and the next day I was flat out. All the symptoms came back. Slowly I began to feel all right again but I noticed that when I went out I could only walk about 100 yards and I felt as though I'd just finished a marathon. I'd come back, sit down and my legs would feel most peculiar. It felt as though I'd got an animal inside me running around from the knees down. My stomach felt as though it was full of electricity. I was so depressed because when you've been very active and you suddenly get low, you feel murderous. Inside you want to do these things but your body won't let you. First I lost weight and then I started to put it on. I put on about two stone because I was so inactive and that worried me because they say if you put weight on you'll have a heart attack and so on. I tried doing a few exercises but I'll tell you now, with M.E. you just can't.

At least I had the sense to know that if I kept it up too long I would make myself worse. Now I don't even go out. If I go out with anybody they've got to walk at my pace and they have to stop every 10/15 yards so I can just lean against a wall or if there's a seat, rest and try to go on again. My daughter, Kim, and I have got round this now. I love going into shops so she takes me to IKEA, the big Swedish furniture shop, where you can hire wheelchairs. As I get out of her car, she puts me in the wheelchair and we spend a few hours wandering around without feeling exhausted; that's a real treat for me.

When I first got M.E. there was a lot of talk about yuppie flu, and every so often there would be some publicity about it. Then Clare Francis spoke about the different symptoms of this yuppie flu on TV and I could have jumped for joy because I thought 'My God, that's the same thing that I've got.' I got so frightened at the beginning because I thought I had a brain tumour because of the headaches. It seemed as though everything had gone wrong in my body.

At the same time as I caught flu and the M.E. began, my daughter, my son-in-law and my grand-daughter all caught it too. Out of all the family there were four of us who had M.E., which left just three who didn't catch it. My son-in-law Ken went down with it, then Mia my granddaughter, and finally my daughter Vanna.

Vanna came round and said, 'I feel so ill and I don't know what's wrong with Ken either. I feel so sorry for him. He's got no energy, he can hardly walk. And Mum, I've always been lazy, I don't like cleaning, but I just can't be bothered to even lift things. I'm getting such terrible pains in my chest. I'm so frightened in case there's something wrong.'

Unlike me, Vanna wanted to know what was wrong. She went to the doctor but that was no use. They thought she was malingering and that it was all in her head. She used to cry to me. She'd say, 'Mum, how can you just think you can't breathe, how can you only think you've got pains and yet you can't walk or anything? Why do they keep saying it's in my mind?' I couldn't help her because I had the same problems. But she's not like me as I ignore these opinions, whereas Vanna has to investigate what's going on. The three of them just deteriorated and no doctor believed her. Eventually she did find a woman doctor who referred her to someone researching M.E. in Cardiff. He's not authorized to advertise that he's researching M.E. because if he did his money would be cut.

When Vanna was attending the hospital she met a friend whose young daughter sat next to Mia at school. The next thing we heard was that this young girl was also very ill with M.E. I wonder if there's a connection, whether it's contagious in the early stages?

I have never been told by a doctor that I have M.E. They can't test you for it. The only way my granddaughter was found to have M.E. was by accident. The three of them – my granddaughter, my daughter and her husband – had been looked at in hospital and were told they were all right. Then, as they were coming out of hospital, my granddaughter had a turn. My daughter rushed her straight back and she had a brain scan. They could apparently see from the scan that there was definitely something wrong. But what happened after that is a mystery, for they then denied they'd said this to her.

They tried a new thing with Mia where they gave her a blood transfusion. She was in hospital for a day and for the following six months she was fine and then gradually her condition deteriorated again.

I think I'm an optimist. I'm going to beat this thing. I'll try anything. I can't just let the world pass me by and not know what's going on out there. I want to be involved and be with the children again. I'm naturally an extrovert and the M.E. has stopped me from doing all the things I've wanted to do. People used to call in here with their troubles and I was able to sit and listen to them for hours, but now I haven't the patience. If they knock, I think, 'oh no, not them'. That's what hurts. I've spent so many hours in this room listening to people who have been in trouble and trying to find ways of helping them, and now I can't face them. I haven't seen Ken, Vanna and Mia for over a year now. They moved to Wales and at first I used to go, but while I was OK in the car on the way there, when I arrived the M.E. symptoms started. And seeing the three of them there with the same illness depressed me. For some reason M.E. makes you lose interest in people. Before, I loved people, I loved talking to them, particularly children.

In 1980 my husband Owen and I helped set up an adventure playground. While we were doing this there were a lot of children just coming out of school and getting into trouble. When they were picked up some were put into homes. We decided that if we got those children into our home, into a family, we could help them. We came up with the idea that we would get them back to school 100 percent and keep them out of trouble. We approached the Head of Intermediate Treatment (IT) at our Council office. We asked how much it cost to put one of these kids into a home. He told us £450 per week, so we asked whether he would be interested if we could do it for £5 a week. I said that we would guarantee that the kids were 100 percent back in school. My son-in-law Ken would help them with their English. Vanna who was very clever with maths would help them with their maths and I'd just give them plain common sense about not getting into trouble. He asked, 'Well, what would you want £5 for?' I said that if they went to school they'd get two weeks' pocket money at the end of the week, which would deter them from stealing. Anyway, he agreed and we had about ten kids here. My husband used to go round all the schools checking them in. Then after school they used to report to us here. Nine times out of ten they would be here till nine or ten o'clock each night because their own home life was terrible. It was a great success. With kids we knew who were sent to the police courts, I'd plead with the magistrate to let them come to us.

In 1979 or 1980 we were told that we couldn't continue with the work. The Head of Intermediate Treatment at the Council left and a new man arrived who didn't like our approach. They simply closed the IT project down. We gave each of the children their bank books and closed. We then concentrated on creating the adventure playground which would encourage kids who need help to congregate. Although officially we were told we could no longer deal with the children, unofficially we just carried on. The kids would still come here, but we couldn't pay them. They would still arrive at the house and stay if they got discharged from Brixton police station; nothing changed much. We still had social workers phoning us up to take the odd child, but we had to turn them down despite their persistence.

In the end, however, the M.E. prevented me from attending meetings and began to affect my involvement with the adventure playground altogether. Lambeth Council will tell you that I was a tough fighter. We really fought for that playground. They didn't want us to have it but I went to all the meetings and battled until we got the site and could build what we wanted. We wanted older play-leaders who the kids would not feel threatened by. They tend to be threatened by play-leaders their own age. Now we have a grandmother as the head play-leader and they can relate to her.

When the M.E. prevented me from being involved, I felt terrible. I was so frustrated. The crime in Stockwell and Brixton is getting worse. At the playground I hung up a banner about drugs and how they screw you up, but the last time we put the banner up the local drug users burnt it.

I know that there is a lot more that I could do around here and I am so angry that my condition has stopped me. My body seems practically finished, but inside there's still the go-getter. Stuck in here, I'm no good for anything and nothing gets achieved. I don't go out anymore. I love reading but that's about all I've managed to catch up on since the illness began. I read anything. I love biographies. I love Jack Higgins. I'm not fussy at all.

When you are well yourself and you see people in wheelchairs, you do momentarily feel sympathy but once they've passed, they are out of your mind. But now, if I see anything on TV about people fighting to have a ramp put in I understand what that fight is about. It's a fight against being stuck, being immobilized, and all the frustration, despair and anger that stems from it.

The best thing that's emerged out of my being ill has been knowing that I have a family who support and believe in me. If you haven't got that, and you're on your own, then it's just someone coming in whose been *told* that you've got M.E. – that makes a difference. I think there are a lot of people with M.E. who are going through what I went through, thinking they've got a brain tumour or cancer, because no one is prepared to diagnose M.E.

The most important thing for me is my family, especially my young daughter Kim. Vanna lives too far away. She's very concerned about me and phones regularly, but I always tell her I'm fine because she is ill herself and worry would make her worse. Kim is very understanding. She never makes me feel guilty. My husband, he's the same, he never pushes, he'll tidy up for me if I don't feel like doing it.

Three years before Kim got married to Martin and I was already ill with M.E., she came into my bedroom and told me that Martin had been shot and was in intensive care. He had to have his spleen removed and three ribs where the shotgun had blasted them, and he had shotgun pellets in his body. His career with the fire service was over. He couldn't carry, he could do nothing. He couldn't even do the job that he'd trained for before, carpet laying, because of carrying and pulling large rolls of carpet. Now he's a mini-cab controller, which he hates. Kim won't let him use the car anymore. She brought him here when he came out of hospital. Nurses visited him at home each day. I suppose Kim brought him here to draw on my experience of being ill. Then when my daughter Vanna was up here before she went to Wales she moved in with me because she was so ill herself. She, Mia and Ken stayed here for six months. Even with the M.E. I felt I *had* to listen to them. And I still give them my sympathy and love whenever they need it.

I've experienced a lot of discrimination, even some of the people that call on me here stare blankly at me when I mention M.E. Take the doctor across the road. Although someone close to her has got M.E., she'll tell you straight that she doesn't understand it. I gave *her* a leaflet!

When the M.E. first started I was in terrible pain with both knees and they were very red and inflamed. I didn't want to go to my doctor, no way, but I thought that if I went, perhaps he would give me something for the knees. The pain in both knees had become so bad that I had to sit down carefully when I bent them. When I mentioned the knees to the doctor, he took a look at them and pressed them. I remarked on the inflammation, the redness, but after he'd prodded them a bit he just sat in his chair, got his pad out and said he thought it was arthritis. I asked if it could be M.E. But all he said was that he'd write a note for me to have an x-ray on the knee. I repeated that I'd been ill with M.E. He only replied, 'There you are,' and handed me the note. He didn't even acknowledge that I'd spoken about M.E., he wasn't even curious.

I felt so angry because had he just asked me, 'ME, what's M.E.?', then I could have gone through the different symptoms, but he was totally dismissive. He didn't want to know. I simply lost my temper, tore up the referral note and never went for an x-ray.

In 1988 my son Roger and his wife wanted to send me for a complete check-up. That, I'm afraid, only annoyed me because I knew that what they wanted was for a doctor to confirm that something else was wrong with me. Every time Roger phones he'll ask again, 'What is this M.E.?' I keep going through it but he just won't listen. His wife got on the phone to me recently, worried, and asked why Roger and I always argue when we meet. I said it was because he makes me feel so frustrated, I want to walk out of the room. He just winds me up so that I feel ill after he's gone. She said, 'I'll tell you something, Mum, he's frightened. He's read about it but he doesn't want to admit that you have got it. As far as he's concerned you are well, you're all right and you're just having a phase.' I said, 'It's a bloody long phase, isn't it, all these years,' and she said, 'Yes, but don't blame him, Mum. I listen to him when he's not talking to you; he is frightened of this M.E.'

Roger came over two or three weeks ago and told me about colonic irrigation which he said he'd look into for me. I thought, if it makes him happy, if he thinks he's doing something, I'll let him look into it. I won't do it but I'll let him look into it.

There are things that I know I won't be able to do again, not with M.E. The community work, for example; having the children and sorting them out, cleaning, things like that. I've attempted walking. Where my daughter Vanna lives in Wales there's a lot of walking. I've tried it but it's no good. As I say, I haven't seen my daughter in over a year now. It's just that I know if I go down there I've got to put on an I'm-all-right face and do some walking. I don't like her to think that I'm as bad as I am.

The effect of the M.E. has, if anything, made my husband Owen and I closer as a couple, mainly because I'm in all the time now. He runs the local youth club twice a week. But it's difficult for him to get out because of his eyesight. He's completely blind in one eye and he's got glaucoma and tunnel vision in the other eye.

I don't see many friends, which might be to do with my indifference when they come round. I just can't be bothered to hold conversations with them. I think I've pushed them away because I just haven't got the energy to deal with them, to think of things to say to them. My daughter Kim comes every day and she'll yap like a little magpie about all that's going on outside. I can sit quietly and listen to her because she knows about the M.E., she knows when to stop and when to start. It's sad because there used to be parties going on here until four in the morning.

Since the incident with my doctor I've not been to any doctors, but I've been reading up on essential oils and this is the one medical treatment I would like to have prescribed. The treatment involves massage, applying different oils for different things – stress, pain or anything. It's called aromatherapy. But this is out of the question because of the cost.

I've tried herbal treatments. The Jamaican herbal tonic made me well for a few weeks. Whether it was me saying to myself, yes, it is doing me good, I don't know, but it did get my appetite back. I've also tried ginseng and garlic tablets but I've never felt any effect with them, although I've not felt worse. I drink only mineral water now as opposed to tap water. I'm so frightened about the water not being pure that I just drink bottled water. My husband gets me that.

I think there has been a little improvement. When I first had M.E. I was really ill. I used to get bad palpitations which made me think I had a dicky heart but I've found out that that's one of the symptoms. Now it's as if I'm convalescing and I'm not sick. If I'm sitting I'm fine but if I've got to go downstairs or go to the toilet then I feel instantly worn out. It's like letting the mud settle – once you start moving it stirs and everything goes cloudy again.

From what I've read, spiritual healing seems to be the most effective treatment for M.E. In fact my husband does healing, so if I get very bad headaches he does this healing on my head. It works just like a prayer and laying on of hands. I don't like to put too much on him though. It's only when things are really bad that I ask him, even though he'd do the healing on me every day if I asked. Healers will tell you that when they give out energy the patient takes it from them. I'm frightened that if I take that energy from him he'll have a heart attack as he's not 100 percent fit himself, and I'd sooner have what I've got than take from him. I think if I could, I'd go to the famous healer, George Chapman. I personally believe that I would then see the end of M.E.

There's a story about a man call Bill Parish, whose first wife died of cancer. He remarried and six months into the marriage it transpired that his new wife had also contracted cancer. She persuaded him to take her to a spiritualist meeting. As he sat in the audience the medium picked him out and said, 'Do you know that you could heal your wife sitting next to you?' He couldn't believe it. She talked him into going to another spiritualist who said, 'Do you know you're a healer?' He listened and took the advice and pursued his vocation as a healer. His first patient was his wife. She was eighty-nine when she passed away and was in her thirties when the cancer was first discovered. Anyway, she outlived Bill. In the meantime he was getting patients. People from all over the world used to go to him. Eventually he passed away and left Peggy Parish, his wife, as the healer. She christened Vanna, the first baby she ever christened. When I was twenty-eight she healed me of pneumonia and pleurisy and TB at St Bartholomew's Hospital. All the doctors used to sit at the back and watch her perform the healing. As a result, they allowed her into the hospital to attend to those patients who wanted her treatment.

My mother was a medium, and the stories she could tell you would make your hair stand up. I believe in spiritualism. I think that if I could find a good healer, if Mrs Parish was still here, she would help me. When I had pneumonia and pleurisy, I went to St Thomas's, and the doctor said to me, 'You've got pneumonia and pleurisy, and one lung is completely fluid, that's why you can hardly breathe. Also you've got a TB germ.' I came home and went straight to Mrs Parish. She sat me in the chair in the sanctuary and said, 'You've got pneumonia and pleurisy and one lung is completely blocked. You've also got a TB germ running rampant in your bloodstream.' I'd not said anything to her, she just repeated what the doctor said. She told me not to worry, everything would be fine. That was in August, and by November I was well.

As far as professional help is concerned I'd say spiritual healing has been the main lifeline for me. I'd like to see this treatment on the National Health. There are a lot of people who believe in it, especially the black community, who are great believers. There are days when I want to give up, when I think, if this is what life's going to be like I'll be glad when it's over. But I realize that I've got to keep fighting. Don't say to yourself, 'I'll prove to them I can do it', and then go out and do a two-mile walk. That's not the answer. You have to work in moderation.

At the beginning I did over exert myself, which is what I think made me more ill. After fourteen days of a flu-like virus, you'd think you'd be on your way to recovery. I still felt very ill but I went back to my job thinking that I ought to be better by now. I did the cleaning, cooking, washing and really wanted to believe that this was the end of it. I felt so tired and I paid for the effort. For the next day or so I was no good to anybody. All I wanted to do was sleep, sleep, sleep. The brain just shuts down. Some say they get attacks of insomnia, but it's the opposite for me. If you can sleep it's the finest healing treatment and the body gradually recharges itself.

My son Roger once bought me an exercise bike. He thought that if I couldn't walk perhaps I'd keep my muscles supple by using the bike. This made sense to me, so each morning I'd have a go. Five minutes would be about all I could manage, and then I'd have to lie flat out for the next five hours. After about three mornings of doing this I noticed that my legs weren't feeling any better. In fact I was getting a sort of jumpy sensation in the muscles during the night. I stuck it for about a week but then I stopped because all the M.E. symptoms came back. I knew then that the bike wasn't for me. It's up on the landing now, waiting for him to take it back. I think yoga is probably the best form of exercise because it's gentle. Common sense tells me that exercise is necessary, but that the gentlest way of moving the muscles and the body is not aerobics or Mr Motivator jumping around, which would kill me.

I should lose weight but I'm not a big eater. In the morning I have half a slice of toast, hardly any lunch, and a very small meal for tea, so I put the weight gain down to lack of exercise. I was so active before, you see, so all the muscles have wasted now.

As far as mobility is concerned, I'm alright if Kim visits with her car. Otherwise it's almost impossible for me to get around. I have used public transport occasionally but often I feel faint, especially if I've stood for a while, then I feel like I'm going to pass out.

I haven't given up on the housework. I am house-proud and I do like my place looking nice. The top of the house I can't manage, so my daughter does that for me. The passage and the kitchen I can cope with at my own pace, as long as everyone's out and I'm left with no one bustling around me. But again I'm lucky, because I've got a daughter who comes in and helps.

Often Owen, my husband, or whoever happens to walk in, has to finish what I've started. Sometimes I look at Owen and I think to myself, he's so lucky to be able to go out and do the things he wants to do. Then I get frustrated and in a temper with him but he's so placid it just flows over him. He looks at me as if to say, 'She's off again, having another wobbly!'

I get occasional bouts of depression because of the general lack of understanding that I have to face. Part of me says they do understand, otherwise I wouldn't get their help and cooperation, and another part says my family are helping just because I'm Mum. I have a doubt whether they really believe that I've got M.E. It's a predicament, because outwardly I don't show any signs of illness, so I feel I have always to explain and justify my condition in case I'm seen as only pretending to be ill.

When I'm depressed I get very tearful. I think to myself, why me? I retreat into myself, and I won't speak to any of the family. I think that hurts them more than me. They'd sooner I shouted at them than do the quiet act. But I'm not doing it to be manipulative – it's just simply how I feel.

I do get myself out of it though. I look at Owen and tell myself that it's not much of a life for him either. He's had a heart attack, he's almost blind, and there's me ignoring him and causing him unhappiness. So I talk myself out of it by feeling sorry for him. I'm the one to blame, not him.

Owen thinks that I've coped well, all things considered. He wishes I'd get out more. He takes the kids to France for day trips or up to Blackpool to see the lights but I won't go anywhere. It's the companionship he misses, someone to talk to and he needs someone to rely on because he can't see very well.

There are so many people who have got M.E. In America alone there are 150,000 cases. Surely that warrants better research into the disease. Think of how many work hours are lost through people who have got M.E., who are pushing themselves to go to work. A nurse I know with M.E. does two shifts a week – she can't do any more – but she has to work because she has children. Funding for research into M.E. should be an absolute priority.

To combat the prejudice I'd campaign as they do for AIDS and multiple sclerosis. I'd campaign for funding through the media. TV is the medium which gets the message to a wide cross-section of people. When you look at something visual the image gets to you.

I think Clare Francis succeeded in cutting through the discrimination against M.E. sufferers because of her star status and because people liked her. The Dean of Westminster, on the other hand, who fought hard for years to reach practitioners and to get them to recognize M.E. as a problem, made little impression on people. Who's the Dean of Westminster? But Clare, she's young, she's known for her sailing and is therefore listened to. There must be other well-known people who have M.E. If they were to come forward and talk about it openly, what could be a more potentially constructive campaign than that?

If I was to give advice to people who have M.E., I would say listen to your own body and know your own limits. Don't stop searching or pushing for different things. There are choices at hand. I think people with M.E. should go to a library and research all the alternative treatments available. That's what I'm going to do. Somehow I'm going to try aromatherapy and see how I get on.

What people should *not* do is to take notice of a doctor who suggests they should see a psychiatrist. Don't listen to people telling you to get out and do this or that exercise. There's been recent speculation that a lot of the additives in food stirs up M.E., which is another thing I'm going to investigate, to see if maybe a change of diet would help. Some days I'm feeling worse than on others but I've never actually bothered to write down what I've eaten each day. I should keep a list and when I feel bad I could look up what I've eaten on that day.

My memory has certainly been affected. I've lost two letters recently that I know I've put away safely. I can be having a conversation one minute and then in the next it's an effort to pick up where I've left off. We've had a relative come over from America recently to trace her roots. I hope she doesn't come to me because the past is such a haze. My daughter Vanna does a similar thing, suddenly in the middle of a conversation it goes all garbled. She calls it 'googly'.

I've got a friend called Joyce and her daughter-in-law Wendy sometimes comes to see me. We'll be having a conversation and I'll attempt to say her name, but it's gone and I'm just left looking at her. I've known Joyce for thirty years, so I feel a total fool. I'd probably forget where I live, but I don't go out!

# Jane Colby

Jane was born in 1945, is a trained dance specialist and former head teacher. She is now a writer, and lives with her son, a research scientist, in Essex.

The way my M.E. started was actually very dramatic, because I can remember the day and even the time of day when it first hit me. I was a head teacher at the time and it was half-term. Ian Gow, the minister for housing had been invited to this big do at the school where he was to open this old people's complex. I can remember standing there in the wind in a pale blue suit, waiting for him because he was late. I had these awful, awful pains across my back, and I thought I was getting flu. When we got back to the school for lunch, these pains had just got worse and worse. Ian Gow sat next to me at lunch because he wanted to talk about children. Questions like, were children any different these days from when I first started teaching, that kind of thing, and I felt worse and worse. That beginning is very clear in my mind but afterwards is almost a complete blank.

This was June 1985. What I can remember about the way my M.E. developed is a bit like little photographs, little images, with the between bits being a complete blank. I think it's partly to do with the fact of it being so dreadful that you block out the memories. I suppose it's rather akin to people saying that you don't remember the pain of childbirth. As far as I know the brain is affected, so this may be the reason why I've forgotten.

I do remember trying to get back to school and feeling like death. I remember one day driving home, and stopping off at the doctor's surgery and arguing with the receptionist, 'You must let a doctor see me today, I'm so ill.' I'd had odd viral infections in the past which were not very pleasant and went on for several weeks and I thought that probably I had another one of these strange viruses. The doctor said 'Perhaps it's Royal Free disease,' which is one of the names that's been given to M.E, so full marks to him for being on the ball.

It then took some weeks to get a proper diagnosis. All through the summer holiday, blood tests showed that I had immune complexes in the blood which meant I'd had some kind of weird virus thing. There had been some research on this, so they cultured the virus out. It turned out to be Coxsackie B, a relative of the polio virus, and I was told, yes, that's what you've got, M.E.

It was Dr Elizabeth Dowsett who rang me at home to tell me. I asked how long it would go on for. I thought she'd say something like a few weeks or so, but she said that in ten years time it'll probably be just a memory. I thought she must be joking. It's now nine years and it's not just a memory. The worst of it is just a memory, but it's my life and everything still has to be organised around the fact that I've got M.E.

That's how it all started. I tried to struggle on with the job for about four years but I had relapse after relapse. I was head teacher of a primary school and it was at the time when teachers were going on strike. The government was getting into some confusion over education and asking us all to produce policy documents which they then later scrapped in favour of a national curriculum. As a result, teachers were refusing to do dinner duties, anything that could have really helped. Everybody always says that the one thing you have to avoid if you want to get better reasonably quickly from M.E. is overwork and overstress.

There was enormous pressure on me and the hours were phenomenal. I would get home and go to bed. I'd ring up supply teachers and have to work in bed. I was in pain all the time. I couldn't think properly. I always had to sit down. When I took assembly I'd talk to children whom I knew perfectly well but I would forget their names. I'd forget the names of teachers too. I would have to have written in front of me what I was going to do or I'd forget. It was appalling.

When I went back into school after the first really bad episode of M.E., I couldn't even walk up the path. I had to get to school by taxi. My mother came with me and actually helped me. She had to support me up the path. I had someone to open the door for me because the doors were too heavy and then I'd have to lie down in my office to open the mail. I would stay there for perhaps an hour or two, knowing that I couldn't possibly walk round the school to see people. Then I'd have to get myself home and back to bed.

The accusations directed at those people who supposedly make themselves ill through too much stress are all too familiar, as is the argument that M.E. is some kind of workaholic burn-out. You don't believe that you can't beat the illness through will-power, so you fight it. I find that a lot of people with M.E. say this, but we're talking about an illness that can last for years. The more you read about will-power and thinking positively, the more you'll believe you can overcome it, but you can't. I should never have struggled into work that ill, I know that now, and I've probably slowed up recovery as a result of doing that. I had four years of struggle, punctuated by constant periods of time off.

My husband, who is a GP, was one of those who found it difficult to believe that I was ill. Because of this, I basically had no one to look after me. I had to stay with my mother. The only reason I could actually carry on with my job was because she did everything else. All I had to do was get out of bed, get to school and back again as soon as I could at the end of the day. She did the washing, the cooking, everything. I did nothing. If I'd had to do anything like that, I could not have carried on with the job as long as I did.

There were times when I thought I would beat it. The National Association of Head Teachers recommended that people who couldn't take a proper lunch hour at the normal time should go off the premises later for a proper break, somewhere where people wouldn't be asking you to do things all the time. I only lived five minutes away, so I used to go home to rest after the official lunch hour. This didn't go down well with the staff, so in the end I stayed at school all day.

In 1989 I had a big crisis from the point of view of my health. I was determined that the school should have it's usual summer concert, so I went ahead and produced it, even though it wasn't as good as it had been in the past when I was fit. You can drive yourself to do things like this with M.E., but what you don't anticipate are the terrible after-effects. I was playing the piano for the finale, I was pouring with sweat, and I felt like death. When the finale was over, I went to my room and collapsed. I was in great pain and my doctor told me to go straight home and get to bed. When I told him we had another concert the next day, he just told me straight that there was no way I could manage it. And that was that. I sat at home and I thought, how ridiculous, there is more to life than dragging your body about and punishing yourself just to try and keep the school up and running, only to drag yourself home finally to bed.

During those four years I'd had a number of crises. On one occasion I was in hospital in the cardiac ward plugged into a heart monitor because I'd had such terrible chest pains. I thought, that's it, I'm coming out of this job. I thought I'd improve straightaway, but I'd run myself so far into the ground, that it took a very long time to improve even moderately after that.

I left the job on that day, which was the end of the summer term in 1989. I just walked out of school and never went back. The worst thing about doing that was leaving loose ends. Normally if you leave a job you sort everything out before you go, you do the filing, you throw away the rubbish, you make sure whoever is taking over from you has all the information necessary, and so on. I had to get my secretary to visit me at home. I wrote copious notes for the existing deputy head – who has since become the head – so that she would know as much as possible about what was going on.

Luckily we did have quite regular meetings, so she wasn't entirely in the dark, but there were lots of personal ongoing projects that she would have needed help with. I would dictate a little bit to my secretary, give her some notes, then have to take a break. I felt breathless just talking, it was exhausting. But I hated leaving a trail of loose ends. As you know, parents do tend to complain about one thing or another, and I had one parent who'd accused me of victimizing her child – one loose end. I didn't like walking away from something like that, but I had no alternative if I was to survive. I didn't let myself get too demoralized by the fact that I had to lose what was a twenty-five-year career which I'd assumed was going to continue until I retired.

I turned to writing but found I couldn't concentrate or sit at the word processor for long, because of all the pain and mental confusion. I would do a bit on the days I felt well enough. But the writing kept me going, and I believed that I could actually make a new career out of it.

It costs me well over £3,000 a year to keep as healthy as I am now, which is reasonably strong. I don't use the word 'better' any more because that word tends to be associated with being cured, which then induces people to ask why I've still got a stick and so on. I've got a stick with a seat attached which I use if I get stuck in a queue at a local shop. Somehow I have to keep enough energy for my writing and to be physically well, and just to cook for myself occasionally; I've got a cleaner, a gardener, and someone to do the washing and ironing. I've installed a radio-controlled garage door. I've had to buy a new car with power steering, automatic gears, all electric, including even a switch to open the petrol cap so the local garage can put the petrol in for me. My whole lifestyle is now designed to be energy-saving. Normally I only need to go upstairs once and that's to bed. For the rest of the day I won't use energy in going upstairs, I save it for writing.

If I have to drive down to the local shops, the repercussions from this often prevent me from working for weeks. I'll have a bit of a downturn because of that, with lots of pain. There just isn't any point in struggling to make yourself active because you just make yourself worse. It's a case of hibernating when that happens and keeping your morale up, making phone calls to friends, writing letters, getting on with your writing and not worrying if you can't get out. I also have most of my shopping delivered once a week. I just pay for everything to be done for me that I can afford and although this is expensive, it does at least mean I've got the strength to do other things. This is the way I have to live.

If I go anywhere, I mean really go anywhere, it's like an expedition to the North Pole. I won't use public transport because of the standing around and the stairs at stations and so on. When I was asked to appear on Kilroy, I said I'd do it if I was sent a car to drive me there and back. I knew if I went on public transport I would be too tired to even speak. I spend about ten to twelve hours a day resting in bed. This usually means that I have to spend quite a bit of the morning in bed otherwise I'd have to in the evening, which is a less normal lifestyle. Most people are around in the evening and if you've gone to bed it's not very sociable. I still need a lot of rest. Some months you feel stronger than others, for no apparent reason. If then I start cutting down on rest, it's all right for a few days. Then slowly you begin to get more and more exhausted. One of the things that's affected is my heart: I get palpitations and tachycardia. I now know that if by just getting out of a chair my heart rate shoots up, then I really must rest.

I'd describe my symptoms in terms of pain and mental fog. I lost a lot of my vocabulary when I was first ill, and said things backwards. I had pins and needles and very peculiar crawling feelings in my skin. My left side was worse affected than my right. At the moment I'm not in pain, which is quite nice, but a lot of the time I am, even if it's only a few little aches and pains. You get so used to it that sometimes you just don't notice it any more. If I try and walk too far it feels as though a sparkler has been set off inside my leg. I get this strange twitching, as if all the fibres in the muscle are contracting independently of each other instead of working together.

The exhaustion goes without saying. I never walk further than I need to because I know what it does to me. Exhaustion is a silly word to use really, I much prefer to use the word weakness, people understand weakness. The muscles go like jelly: you tell them to grip something and there's just nothing there, as if you can't control them. It is a real weakness that is generalized throughout the muscles.

When I was first ill I had to pull myself upstairs with my arms because my legs weren't working properly, and in order to comb my hair I had to rest my elbow on the dressing table just to be able to lift the comb to my hair. Even these days, when I dry my hair it hurts to hold the hairdryer up, I have to keep passing it from one hand to the other in order to rest the muscles.

I have a lot of temperature problems. I'll get too hot or too cold, irrespective of what the temperature is. I also have to eat regularly, even if it's only small amounts, because if I don't I get very disorientated and feel very peculiar, a bit like somebody who's got low blood sugar. I find that certain smells now give me headaches where they didn't before – fumes, say. A chap came to mend the television once, and I suddenly realized that because he was doing some soldering I would have to open all the windows and doors and get outside. That still happens. Sometimes it will be a perfume that makes me feel sick. Certainly anything like paint, or solvents that you find in pens, make me feel a bit dizzy and odd.

I have had to change dentist a number of times until I found somebody who was prepared to use a particular injection that does not have adrenalin in it because otherwise I tend to faint. The first dentist used to say silly things like 'Oh, you're just het up, dear...' which was exceedingly irritating. I'd been going to that dentist for years and years, and even though I know that at a dentist you have a tendency to get a bit uptight, I'd certainly never had a problem like that before. Because of not being able to have an ordinary injection, I do feel some of the work that's being done, but it just about stops me from jumping around. I've even had pins put in a tooth with no anaesthetic at all because of the fact that the chap I was going to at the time didn't have one without adrenalin, so I chose to have nothing. It wasn't pleasant but I didn't feel ill, I had no after-effects. When I have an injection I daren't drive to the dentist because I might run into something on the way back. I always take a taxi as even small amounts of local anaesthetic make me feel very woozy.

I have mood-swings, although they're less bad than they used to be. Initially I became easily upset about absolutely nothing, and it was only after a while that I realized I was suddenly feeling depressed or miserable or even euphoric for no reason at all. It just happens, it's something you're not able to control. It seems to happen because of something chemical in the brain. It's not related to anything that's going on or to any stress. This does mean, though, that you're very much more vulnerable to anything happening around you, and that can provoke an exaggerated response from you. I don't find that's nearly so bad as it used to be; it's got a lot better. Also it's partly because I've got used to what might happen. I still have bouts of tachycardia – very, very rapid heartbeat – and that's very frightening. You can also have panic attacks with M.E. I have had these attacks but now I can recognize the early signs and can generally control them.

I've had very bad problems with my intestines, a bad stomach, and at the moment I sleep most of the night propped up on my pillows, not lying flat, because I find it's just easier on my gut that way. I've got used to it. I may wake up at about six in the morning, put the pillow down and go to sleep for another couple of hours lying flat, but most of the night I'm partly propped up. I had to do that when I was pregnant and had bad indigestion, it's the same sort of thing. What tends to happen though is that you mask the fact that you're still getting these symptoms because you're learning to cope with them and you can stop them happening through modifying your lifestyle. But if you tried to live the way a normal person would live, the symptoms would all come back again. That's one of the points that needs emphasizing, because people see me at the shops when I'm looking okay and what they don't see is the time in between when I can't get out and about. In view of this, it's hard for people to believe that there is something seriously wrong.

I used to work myself hard because I loved my job. I've always been very active. When I was a baby my mother said I ran before I walked, and I think that's the way I've approached life. I was a squash player, I loved to dance, and the dance training I did was similar to ballet training, very hard physical work. I've done rock climbing and mountain walking, and at school there was always some project going on. I loved working with children and when I became head teacher I produced a lot of shows and that kind of thing. The most frustrating thing after I got M.E. was that I still had the urge to do all these things, it didn't go away. The moods of depression, the tiredness and exhaustion, the pain, never stopped me from wanting to do things and the frustration was indescribable. I think one of the most important things I had to learn was that while I'm basically a different person it doesn't mean I won't be able to do things I enjoy or to achieve new things – they will just have to be things that come within the scope of someone whose body has got M.E.

I'm very positive most of the time. Occasionally I'm not because I might watch something on television which will bring home to me the way I used to be able to dance and I might have a good cry about it. Some things occasionally frighten me, such as the possibility of never being any fitter than I am now. I think to myself, what happens if, before I eventually end up being able to support myself through writing, or if for some reason I never do, they start cutting State benefits, what on earth shall I do? I will be really poor and what then? I won't be able to afford my housekeeper, or this and that, and I know that as a result I'll get seriously ill.

People have committed suicide with M.E. and I can understand how in a severe depression you'd come to that. I can also understand doing it from knowing that you'll never be any better. Being poor as well as having to look after yourself is a vicious circle in terms of this illness and I can understand why someone would want to be out of it.

I don't like to be socially isolated because I think it's bad for me. I can't see people a lot but I make phone contact. I'm often on the phone to someone or other. I don't always like to write about M.E., because again I want to be as normal as possible. I like to write on different subjects. The novel I'm writing is a thriller. M.E. is the one subject that if I am asked to write something knowing I'm not going to get much of a fee I'll still do because I think it's important to get the information across. For other subjects I demand a sensible fee, but I wouldn't only want to write about M.E. It's not healthy to dwell entirely on the thing that has so much impact on my life, and I want to have as normal and healthy a life as I can within those limits.

M.E. is a disability and so I share a lot of the problems with other disabled people in society. I've got a very good friend who goes all over the place with me and recently it was suggested that I might like to go round Costco which is a huge supermarket. I said that I would be quite interested but that we'd have to take the wheelchair. Although he's pushed me around in the wheelchair before now, he said on this occasion, 'You don't want to be seen in that.' I remember his words because they upset me and made me angry. Fit people wouldn't be seen dead in a wheelchair and of course there is this awful stigma attached to them. But it makes me very cross. If I travel by plane, which isn't very often, I use their wheelchair facilities without fail because airports are huge and with M.E. you suffer. I could walk that distance if I really pushed myself but then I'd be ill for the rest of the week on holiday. There's no point in that, so I use their wheelchair facilities and am not ashamed to use them.

When you first realize that you are disabled you're upset because you are part of a society that is prejudiced against the disabled. It's only when you become disabled that you realize how prejudiced *you* were before. You've got to accept the fact that you are disabled, you've got to overcome your own shame at being in a condition based on your original prejudice, and then you've got to learn to integrate these concepts into a new attitude towards society in general.

I think I have become a better person through this experience, because I think I've got a much more enlightened view of people who use wheelchairs since having to resort to one myself. I don't enjoy being disabled or being pushed around but at the same time I don't get so upset about it any more. When a photographer came to photograph me for an article recently that I did for *Disability Now*, he said, 'We may have to move the furniture around.' I said, 'Well, you do that, I'm not going to make myself ill.'

I very rarely go far because I don't have anyone to drive the car for me and it exhausts me to drive too far. If I could pay for a chauffeur I'd be out much more, but I am not going to wear myself out and then find I can't do my writing. You've got to concentrate on priorities with M.E. If writing is what I want to conserve my energy for I'm not going to waste it driving to a town ten miles away. I order my clothes by mail. I can't walk around a supermarket so someone else has to go for me, most stuff I buy locally anyway. You make life choices based on the necessity to conserve energy because you know you haven't the resources that other people have. If I was still using all my energy and time running a school, I wouldn't be writing, which is one positive result of having M.E. and also a life-long ambition fulfilled. So in a way, as one door closes, another opens.

One of the things that Dr Darrell Ho-Yen says in his book, *Better Recovery from Viral Illnesses*, is that people become acutely aware of their own frailties. They have to face up to themselves, as opposed to those who spend their lives avoiding such decisions and not having to think about things. I wish I'd seen that book when I first got M.E. because I had to work it out for myself, needing to reorganize my life, keep a diary about what did or did not make me worse, so that I could report to doctors if necessary. Dr Ho-Yen finds that patients who go along with his advice do best and I seem to have independently worked towards the advice that he gives. I've talked to him about something I was writing on sex and M.E., and we had a good laugh. It's impossible for someone who hasn't got M.E. to really know what it's like, yet he was very understanding.

I think M.E. is a bit of a one-off in the sense that you live with the unexpected all the time, you don't know what's going to happen to you from one day to the next. You gradually lose confidence in your body's ability to behave normally because it doesn't, you can't predict what's going to turn up next, so you have to learn to tolerate uncertainty in everything.

If I go somewhere on holiday I have to be very careful in choosing where I go. I have to check out what all the facilities are first in case of a crisis. I didn't take these precautions to start with, and once when I was travelling on a train with my mother, I felt so appallingly ill that when we finally got to the station I collapsed. These awful unexpected things happen, so I'd say that what is most unexpected about M.E. is that you have to learn to live with the unexpected all the time.

There is a funny side also. Action for M.E. has a magazine called *Interaction*, and there is a little section where people report the daft things they've done. Somebody once opened her fridge and found a shoe instead of the butter. I'm reminded of those lovely cartoons that Martin Arber's wife, Yvonne, does. He's the editor of *Interaction* and this came up when I was doing the article on sex and M.E. One of the cartoons depicted a woman saying to a man 'Oh, darling, you haven't forgotten where you're up to again, have you?' Another is of a woman at the doctor's saying, 'Yes, I can manage foreplay now, and intercourse, but I have to have a week's rest in between.'

You have to overcome all kinds of embarrassment with M.E. I was taken quite ill in London in a theatre one afternoon, with tachycardia which went on for ages and I was exhausted with it. In the evening, we were eating in a carvery and I said to my friend, 'You'll have to go and get the wheelchair, I can't get back to the room without the wheelchair.' 'I can't bring that wheelchair in here, there's no room between the tables,' he said. I insisted, so fair enough, he went and got it. As we were pushing our way through, there was a whole queue of people staring studiously ahead to avoid looking at me, you know the way people do, I looked at them and said 'Mind your backs,' which broke the ice. Often an embarrassing situation can transform into an amusing one.

The foremost thing that comes to mind in terms of achievement is I had to learn what I wanted to write. I found that I was studying other people's books in a way I hadn't before. I've read all of Dickens since I've been ill which is an achievement. I read new novels, which encourages me to find my own way of writing. My own style is an achievement. One day I might write short stories in a feminist style. I'll write another way if I want to write an article about issues like disability. I can turn to a more academic style or to something which is perhaps more chatty, and there's also this novel which I'm determined to get published one way or another. That will be an enormous achievement as it's so hard to get a first novel published. A publisher doesn't like taking risks with unknown authors. But since I've begun writing I go on achieving. The first achievement was to get something published, the second was to get paid for it and the next was an editor who said he liked my work so much he wanted me to write for him every month and would I like to use my own ideas.

I can go on writing for as long as I'm fit, and I have every intention of doing so. I'm as ambitious now as I ever was, it's just a shift in direction. The frustrating thing is that I'm aware of the limitations of what I can do now. But this has enabled me to learn to use the resources I do have. If I'm doing an article about something, I collect lots of information and put it in a file over a period. Eventually, when the first line comes to me, I'll sit down and write that article with all the bits and pieces of information in front of me and I'll find that my brain has been quietly working away on its own, so I haven't had to spend all the time sitting at the word processor. My brain has done some of that work for me already without me being conscious of it. I've developed a conscious system of working, whereby I collect bits of information, put them aside under the heading that I want to write, and so by the time I go back to it the work is half done.

The problems that I've come up against have been to do with the medical profession. The doctor who first diagnosed me was absolutely excellent for a time. He gave me some bad advice on a couple of occasions but I put this down to not knowing enough about the condition. I did say once that I felt a lot better and asked if I should go back to playing squash. He told me that if I felt up to it then there was no reason why I shouldn't give it a go. I ended up in hospital because I was taken so ill afterwards.

Another doctor prescribed me beta-blocker drugs because of the palpitations and the tachycardia. I didn't like taking them because my limbs used to go dead. I would wake up and find parts of my body completely dead and the beta-blockers seemed to make it much worse. On one occasion the doctor wouldn't come out, but told my mother over the phone to give me another beta-blocker, whereupon my blood pressure dropped so low that an ambulance had to be called. I was plugged in to a heart monitor all night. My heart rate was 38/45, very low. I had taken too much of this drug. I was really angry about what happened but was too ill to pursue it.

Another time I had a very bad dose of flu, another attack of tachycardia, and in general was feeling terrible. I rang up the doctor and asked him to come out for a visit. He responded by saying, 'Of course you feel terrible, lying there all the time doing nothing.' I couldn't believe my ears, he'd been such an ally for so many years, and then he said, 'Perhaps you should try and push yourself through the pain barrier. If you find you can walk for twenty yards, well then try one hundred yards and then try half a mile.' I felt so angry and betrayed that the next day I changed my doctor. But to a certain extent I forgive him because I think he'd read one of Simon Wessley's articles, who believes that there probably is a viral reason for the illness but has gone on record as saying that the reason M.E. persists is more to do with the patient's attitude than the original viral cause.

Anybody with M.E. will tell you that if they could they would because they don't need motivation. But I'm much more forgiving than I used to be over these things. It's exhausting to be bitter and unforgiving so there's no sense in it. The doctor I have now is practical and sensible and I believe he knows that if I could I would. My worst times have been fighting against these prejudices.

The only thing I didn't manage to overcome was cooking for myself. Most of the time I eat frozen or instant food, and now I won't burn up energy even peeling a potato, standing or sitting. If it was my hobby and I loved it then I would, but I would not be able to do anything else. I have to make a choice. For a time I could hardly even open a can. I applied for the benefit to pay to have someone in to cook meals. I was told over the phone that I'd got it but then in writing I was told I hadn't. There had been some mix-up but I was too ill to fight it and there was no one to fight for me. My son was away at university, so I had no alternative but to let that go. The battles I've had have mostly been with benefit agencies and medical practitioners.

When you are in the first, what is called the toxic phase of M.E., you do wonder if it will always be like that, if you'll ever walk down your garden path again and so on. I used to play the piano but I can't play any more, so I sold the piano and bought a hi-fi because I wanted to be able to listen to music again. It used to be very painful listening to dance music and not being able to dance any more, but once I'd made the decision to get rid of the piano the hurt was easier to deal with and I was able to listen again.

I probably read more than I used to as well as taking up writing. I've made a lot of network contacts too. One thing that's completely new and I would never have done without M.E., is the research that Dr Elizabeth Dowsett and I are doing between us to find out about the numbers of cases of M.E. in schools. We started in Essex, and I got the education authority interested in cooperating so that we could use their internal mail system, which made it a very cheap operation. We've covered Essex, Humberside, and we're just about to move on to Hertfordshire, in the hope that all sorts of other authorities will get involved. We're looking at an increasing number of cases of M.E., including staff, and we're finding clusters that exist in schools. I suspect that there are many cases that go unseen. I would say that there's probably about a third of so-called school-phobics who are turning out to be M.E. cases and I wouldn't be surprised if there was a case in every school.

When you run a school you have a network of educational friends but they tend to be in one geographical area. I've now got people I would call friends spreading from Scotland to the Channel Islands to all over the place, just because of this work I've done with M.E. Half of them I've never seen but there's always an invitation to visit them if I can. I met someone for the first time in Guernsey last year who has M.E. herself. It was lovely to meet her and we've stayed in contact by phone for two years. I have, though, lost a lot of old friends, what you would call real fair-weather friends, who only want to know you when you are fit and well and don't know how to relate to you once you've become disabled.

I also use opportunities now in a way I wouldn't have done previously. After I did the Kilroy programme, I told Robert Kilroy-Silk that I was no longer a head teacher but a writer and asked him for an interview. He agreed and was very kind and supportive. We did a phone interview for a magazine. You have to use these occasions.

The research I'm doing won't be completed for possibly another two years because we aim to study as many counties as we can. When we released some results from Essex we got a lot of local as well as national interest. I did a phone-in programme for the radio. I would like to do more publicity for M.E., either on radio or television. With the Kilroy programme I'd planned it so carefully that I actually got away with not having a relapse afterwards. I phoned the hotel to make sure that my room was on the ground floor, and I accepted their offer of a wheelchair so that I could save my energy for the programme.

There are things that I won't attempt to do any more. For instance, the other day I gave away my squash gear and my racquets because I have accepted that I won't be playing squash again.

The other thing I know I couldn't do again is rock climbing, but I'd still love to be able to get up on to a mountain somewhere. I'd like to abseil down from a helicopter or something like that, as long as the drop wasn't from too great a height, to raise money for M.E. I know that physically it's possible if all you have to do is get yourself down, although I would be using a lot of energy. Physically I think I could do something like that now. The only reason that I haven't so far, is that I'm worried about inducing a relapse due to the adrenalin. Even a normal healthy person would probably experience a surge of adrenalin from abseiling off a drop and it's the adrenalin that would push me into a relapse quicker than anything. It's a shame, because I think with enough sponsorship and enough publicity you could raise the profile of M.E. At the same time an event like this could be misinterpreted by those who'd see an M.E. sufferer abseiling down from a height as not having much wrong with her.

One of the biggest questions to address is do you live with someone or not if you're in a relationship. I'm not in a position to be making that decision at the moment but I do wonder about it. My marriage didn't just break up after twenty-one years because of M.E. It had never been a particularly good marriage, and I think that the separation would have happened anyway when our son turned eighteen, instead of it being precipitated by my being ill. But because I had M.E. and couldn't do anything for myself, I decided that I had to move to my mother's just to be looked after.

I've since heard of people who have moved out of the matrimonial home, not because they couldn't get on with their partner, but because it seemed necessary to be free of the responsibilities their immediate family imposes in order to begin to get fit. Dr Charles Shepherd in his book, *Living with M.E.*, points out that it's preferable to live with someone, simply because it's hard to have an emotional relationship if you're constantly saying good-bye. But people have different views on this. I do get lonely, but it's not often.

I've been divorced since 1990 but I haven't lived with my husband since 1985, which was the year when I became ill and we separated. My current relationship is affected in practical ways, such as what we can actually do together. If he suggests a sunny holiday, for example, I know from the outset that I can't cope with the heat or sun. I have to wear sun-glasses, a sun hat, sit in the shade, and drink continuously otherwise I get excruciating headaches and become exhausted. M.E. restricts what you can do and I think that as far as a relationship is concerned, to live with somebody, these considerations have to be understood before such a commitment is undertaken. In most cases, though, people move in together and don't think about their individual needs, or who they really are.

I honestly don't know whether I would prefer to be living with a partner or not. My son, Mark, lives with me but he's twenty-four and a research scientist with his own life. At the moment I can watch whatever I like on television, I can lie about when I like, I can tidy up when I want to, I can get up when I want to, I can eat when I want to. I'm not saying that if I was living with someone I'd have to suddenly run about and transform my existence, but there would be two people to consider. My son doesn't expect me to do things for him, so we're like flatmates.

Mark has helped tremendously from time to time in practical ways. When I was asked to give a lecture on M.E., he took time off to drive me there, otherwise I would not have been able to do it. He also helped me with the overhead projector when it broke and commandeered one from another room. He was then about twenty-two. He's practical and sensible. If I'm ill in the night he doesn't panic, he just phones the doctor or helps me through it. He is not a panicker and therefore marvellous to have around if I'm really ill. But he's got his own life and so it's inevitable that eventually he'll move out or move away. I don't want to burden him by making him feel that he ought to be doing this or that for me, which is not what our relationship is about. I would help him if he needed it and I could, and he would do the same for me. We have a good friendship.

My mother lives near me now. She's seventy-eight and fitter than me. She will ring up and ask if I'd like some letters posted or offer to go to the shops for me. She often makes me Sunday lunch which is rather nice but I like to be independent as much as I possibly can be. She had to do everything for me in the first few years and it was very hard for her to suddenly have to adjust and take on that caretaking role again. She must worry sometimes about what will happen if she gets ill and needs support, and how much can I do for her.

I moved in with my mother when at first I was unable to cope with the M.E. Some of the furniture and stuff was brought over but it was hard for me even to get back into the house to sort out a few clothes. I've got almost no memory of it at all other than that it happened suddenly while I was in hospital and very ill. I had a long session with the doctor who asked me where I would be going once I left the hospital. He knew how difficult things had been with my husband anyway and I thought he'd expect me to say that I would stay with my mother for a while. As it happened that is what I said and what I did. When my husband rang up and asked if I was coming back, I told him that that was the end of it. It wasn't really what you'd call a move but I stayed with my mother for about five years until the divorce finally came through, and I had enough money to buy this little place.

Initially it was horrendous because I owned nothing except a small amount of furniture. I didn't have a cooker. I didn't have any pots or pans, not even a knife and fork. It was like setting up home right from scratch. Somehow I had to find the energy to choose wallpaper and so on. I got some things by mail order. But I pushed and pushed myself too much, so that about two weeks before the move, I was flat out and unable to do a thing.

When it came to the actual move, I had to be moved along with the furniture. I had drawn all these plans of where the furniture should go. My son supervised the move and my mother helped the removal men, who were really quite good. I lay on a couch which was eventually moved, but I can't even remember being driven from one house to the other because I felt so queer. I think it took me a year to get over the move. I don't just mean emotionally – physically it took me a year to get back to where I was. That was 1991.

When I was diagnosed with M.E. I suppose I felt that at least I'd now got something identifiable that had a name. I wasn't surprised it turned out to be viral. If I'd been told I had MS or cancer or some terminal illness, I would have had all kinds of preconceptions to deal with. But I'd never heard of M.E. and so didn't have any preconceptions, which is why I got such a shock when Dr Dowsett said that in ten years' time it might just be a memory. I thought she was joking. I didn't know then that M.E. was a disability. I understood it to be a viral illness that would just go away. I didn't realize that most people – I think, 75 percent – who get M.E. do end up with some degree of permanent disability.

The same would apply to MS. It wasn't a nasty shock in the way it would have been if I'd been told I had something I already knew to be very serious. But because I didn't know what M.E. really was, like a lot of people, I had to find out what it meant. I did a lot of research on the condition. I wanted to find out as much as I could. And then it gradually dawned on me that it was going to be a very long-term thing and that my whole life would change as a result. It was a long and gradual realization, finding out what M.E. meant.

People ring me about their children who've got M.E. They're worried in case the children drop behind with their school work. I say that the first thing they have to accept is the fact that the average case lasts four and a half years and that they're likely to be in for a long haul. There's nothing they can do about this. No amount of fighting is going to alter the condition. You might be lucky and it could last only a few months if you let the child rest enough now. It's alarming being faced with news like this. But then I've also had people get back to me who've said that I helped them realize that their child's health is more important than whether he passes an exam. It was the same for me too – only when I realized what M.E. meant could I begin to come to terms with it. The best advice I was given at the time was to modify my lifestyle, which is what I've done.

I haven't really looked into alternative medicine much because M.E. is so variable. The danger of trying a new treatment is that if you get worse you assume it's the treatment; likewise, if you get better you assume the treatment has helped you recover. But M.E. shifts the whole time and invariably adjustments happen anyway. The only way to tell if a particular treatment works is to ensure a proper trial of it. Somebody told me about evening primrose oil. I tried one capsule and had a violent allergic reaction to it. I tried it for about four days, and within about 30 seconds of taking each capsule my stomach gurgled, I had excruciating pains with diarrhoea, and everything. My whole body was trying to reject the thing. Sometimes I take a few vitamins, vitamin C each morning in case I'm a bit short of that. Otherwise, I just modify my lifestyle.

If you talk about diet as treatment, I have had to modify my diet just to avoid things I know will upset me. I can't take alcohol, for example, it upsets my heart rhythm. If I have a glass of wine in the evening, by the following morning my heart rhythm has speeded up and makes me feel peculiar. I don't eat chocolate or cheese or drink coffee. I get awful headaches if I eat chocolate or cheese. I have had the odd migraine since having M.E., which I'd not experienced before, so I avoid the foods that precipitate headaches.

I'm not into alternative treatment at all. I won't even take painkillers unless I've got a really bad headache because I could then be taking them for three months at a time to try to ease the really bad viral pain in my muscles. I am sensible. If I get pains that go on and on, I will go to the doctor and ask him to check me out. He's careful and conscientious, but then he'll always say, 'Yes, viral pains, no treatment.' He's ever so sensible and nice. On the whole I just rest and ignore the pains if I can, unless they are too bad and then I avoid what makes them worse. I find that if I type too much it makes my arm pains worse, which is annoying when I'm trying to write. But I have to be sensible and practical about the whole thing.

I don't use public transport. When you have M.E., you must have everything planned, and working things out on public transport can go wildly wrong. It's true that a car can break down but I carry a phone with me in case it does. I have a friend who went on a train journey and the train broke down. She hadn't anything to eat or drink with her, which made her feel ill, and after about two hours they got everybody out of the train and made them walk into the station. She had a relapse for about two weeks as a result, she was in a dreadful state.

I would travel on public transport if I could get somebody to come along with me in case something happened and to push my wheelchair – and if I knew I could find lifts at the station, wouldn't have to manage all those stairs, and wouldn't have to lift my case. It would be necessary to have someone with me to make sure we got off at the right station and if, say, the doors jammed, to sort that out. One of the most exhausting things is actually making decisions, so if something happens that's out of the ordinary, you really want someone to sort it out for you. If you have to find an official or somebody to deal with it, that means a walk to find them in the first place. You've got to explain what's wrong and so on which all requires energy. Not only have you got to explain that something's wrong, but you've also got to explain that you're ill. The whole thing, which most people just take for granted, becomes some enormous event. I won't go anywhere in general unless I'm chauffeur-driven door to door.

I'll fly only if I can use the care flight system, which means that as soon as you get to the check-in desk, you don't even have to manage your own baggage. Usually there's someone who will help you with that arrangement if you phone through to the airport and then get the wheelchair right the way through. They are very good at looking after you. Everything else we've booked in advance. When I thought I might use a ferry I rang the ferry company. If you let them know when you book the ticket, there are special considerations made for disabled people, special lifts, getting you on to the ferry first, putting you near the lifts with your car, all sorts of things. But you can't just turn up and expect this treatment without prearranging it first; people need to be programmed.

I got myself one of the orange disabled badges for when I travel. I used to be ashamed of being disabled and wearing a badge, but on a journey once, I found that we had to park miles from the loo in a motorway service station. I staggered up the car park and found dozens of disabled spaces right next to the loo. At that point I thought to myself, what a bloody fool, being so proud and ridiculous, we could have parked in one of those. I suddenly realized how very stupid I was being, for I was actually disabling myself. It's when you accept your condition, and ask for everything that's going and are not ashamed to do so, that you might actually get over the journey and still be in some reasonable shape when you arrive at your destination.

A friend of mine was supposed to be on her way to America but the plane got held up and she had a long wait at the airport. Eventually she went home because she realized that from waiting she'd become so ill, there was no point in going. There's a girl who lives in the village here who went to America for a family holiday. She had the most terrible jet-lag, I don't know how long the holiday was but I think it took her a week to get over the journey there, and a week to get over the journey back. You have to remember that travelling is exhausting even for healthy people.

I have someone in to do the housework. I don't do anything. I wipe the top when I've made a few crumbs but my cleaning lady does everything. I won't wash anything during the week when she's not coming because it means I've got to hang it on the line or hang it up or go upstairs to hang it on the airer. I used not to mind doing it, but I soon twigged that it meant I had less energy for my writing. She does all the washing and puts it on the line for me in the morning.

I think M.E. has made me angrier but I've always been a natural rebel. I suppose it's just something else to rebel about. I get angry with my body for mucking my life up. I never used to understand this 'Why me?' business, but what really strikes you when you're ill with M.E. is that you can't comprehend how the world keeps working. You look out and the milkman is doing his rounds, the postman is walking about, and you think, suppose everybody got M.E., nothing would happen, and thank God they're not all like me. Martin Arbor, editor of *Interaction*, says he feels envious of those who can choose to do what they want. My anger is no longer directed towards being disabled, it's at a society which is basically set up to discriminate against people who are disabled and not just with M.E.

The most unhelpful advice has been medical. The recommendations are still based on progressive exercise. As you go through the years with M.E. you learn to trust yourself and what your body is telling you. As a trained dancer I know what it feels like if you've got unfit muscles, and it's the same with walking up mountains or anything that's strenuous. If you've got unfit muscles and you start to exercise them it's actually quite pleasant as long as you don't push yourself too far. But when you have M.E. and you try to walk too far, it isn't just that your muscles feel weak or that they behave in this odd way, which is best described as a twitching sensation. You also feel a central loss of energy. It's like having a black hole in the pit of your stomach, a really peculiar sensation because there is just nothing to call on. If you were to listen to your body you'd know you shouldn't be doing what you're doing. If you've read one of these articles that says you should carry on regardless, you're inclined to doubt yourself, especially if it's doctors who are giving the advice. I think your own body will tell you what's right.

Emotionally I think I've coped bloody well. I've had downturns but determination has pulled me through as much as anything. I've needed the support of other people and although I live mainly on my own at the moment I know that my mother and my son are here. I know that my friend will help me with my needs as well. But I never feel wholly secure. You have to find a way of coping emotionally while knowing that you are insecure. You soon realize that in fact security is an illusion and that life just isn't secure. It's not the human condition to be secure.

People I know have said that they wouldn't have been able to cope in the way that I have. But I say that's nonsense, because you either cope or you go under. It's one or the other, there really isn't the choice. Without sounding vain, a lot of people have said to me they think I've coped extraordinarily well and been very brave. I hate that business, I mean bravery doesn't really come into it because it is a case of choice. Are you going to cope and come to terms with this, or aren't you? You don't know what you might be able to do in the future until you look for it. Coming to terms with M.E. is a case of finding a new way of being, you're just not able to be the same person you were before.

Sometimes I dream that I'm running and I'm running downhill through grass or down a hillside and it's the most wonderful sensation. I remember dancing consciously, but I don't usually dream about dancing. I remember last summer when I was in Guernsey, just for a little experiment I did run a few steps down a hill just to see what it felt like. In my experience you have to listen to your body. I get up sometimes and want to get out to the shops and when I do I know I can walk at a normal pace and anybody looking at me wouldn't know I've got M.E. But those are rare days when I know I can do it and enjoy doing it, but I wouldn't be stupid enough to try and run.

When my divorce was going through I came up against the fact that I had to ask for enough money out of the settlement to buy a house because I couldn't get a mortgage. There was also the question of maintenance and my husband brought up the fact that I might like to insure myself against having to stop work. That was before I stopped work, but I already had M.E. and I found that I couldn't get that sort of insurance. I already had one insurance which is in fact paying out now. It's not index-linked and the payments are going down and down all the time.

It was my husband's lawyer who predictably brought up the fact that I would probably be entitled to benefits. I had a medical which I passed and I got invalidity benefit. I found I was also entitled to things like orange badges, but my own doctor said that I might be eligible for mobility allowance because I couldn't walk very far. I had an examination and was asked to walk about a bit, tested on what I could and couldn't do. I passed the examination but they only awarded the allowance for something like two years. If you didn't agree with the assessment, then you had to object within a certain period of time.

At that time I still couldn't accept the fact that in two years I would still need mobility allowance, so I thought two years, fine. Of course I now realize that this was ridiculous. I was going to have to get a completely different car. I had a car which was almost new, only a few thousand miles on the clock, but with such heavy steering I knew I had to change the thing. I realized that I was going to need mobility allowance from that point of view and also due to the fact that I couldn't get anywhere without the car because of having to park as near as possible to places and through not being able to walk very far. The problem with M.E. is that there are days when you can't walk at all, there are days when you can do a little, there are days when you can do a lot, and there are days when you do too much and you push yourself. It's so variable. Eventually I did appeal and I won. They said it would be open-ended but in fact it runs out in 1996.

Then the whole system changed, and I had an absolutely terrible ordeal with the benefits agency over the new disability living allowance. They were so late in issuing me with a certificate that showed that I was entitled to mobility allowance that I couldn't use it to buy my car, which I should have been entitled to. The last time I had a medical the doctor wrote something I totally disagreed with. My GP also disagreed with the report, so if that ever comes up again there'll be one hell of a fight. It was some ludicrous assumption that he made about being able to go back to work – which sounded as if I was almost better.

We are not talking about people who are going through the very early stages of the illness in that they are so ill that they can't do anything at the time. Suppose they took away my mobility allowance so that I could no longer afford to pay for my car, or took away my orange badge so that I couldn't park on a double yellow line next to a shop or whatever. What would happen is that I would either be totally restricted and have to stay in the house, or I would struggle out and get ill again. As soon as that happens I qualify for benefit again, which is all total bureaucratic madness. I think it's absolutely appalling.

Somebody with M.E. has got to know their limitations. I opted out of counselling people. I did a little and I was also asked to chair some meetings, which exhausted me so much that I felt what I was doing was of limited use. What I do now is write articles and do phone-ins so long as I can manage to do it without making myself ill. Sometimes you take a risk because you think it's important enough. I think it's important to raise awareness when you get the opportunity.

I am also campaigning in schools. This is because I was a head teacher anyway, but I've produced guidelines which were issued first by Essex Education Authority. Now this data automatically goes out to schools taking part in the school survey that we are doing. Action for M.E. has adopted them and we're now into the second edition. I get written to for copies from all over. I also get written to by chief education officers, chief education psychologists, home tutors, and people with hospital and home tutoring units. All kinds of people in education write to me, partly because of the articles I've written in education journals and so on.

Discrimination I think is made up of both ignorance and prejudice. Some people are prejudiced even when they are well informed. I think it's necessary to portray M.E. sufferers as people who aren't wingers or victims, trying to scrounge benefits. I use language in the best way I can. I've written articles on M.E. and sex, M.E. in school children, M.E. and exercise. I've had proposals published in magazines for things like M.E. and the autumn term, M.E. and coming back from holiday. If I can think of some useful peg to hang an M.E. story on, then I will, it's become my specialist area.

One of Her Majesty's Inspectors of Schools, Stewart Robertson, has supported the guidelines and the research. He encourages education authorities to join the survey. He once gave a talk on school libraries and wanted to link it with M.E. Many school children suffer from M.E. and I talked to him about the sort of book that should be available. I'm hoping to do a children's book on M.E. myself because although there is a beautiful leaflet for younger children and there's something like Darrell Ho-Yen's book for older secondary school children and adults, there's a gap in the middle which I would like to fill.

The advice I would give to an M.E. sufferer would be to accept what's happened to you because you can't do anything until you've made that step. There's a lovely Irish statement, 'If I were you I wouldn't start from here.' I'm half Irish myself, and if I was me I wouldn't start from here, but I've got to and I think that's what everybody with M.E. has to remember, that they have to start from where they are. What they shouldn't do is make excuses for themselves, which is the worst thing. People feel guilty that they can't do things and so they try and do them and make themselves ill. The more they feel guilty about things they can't do, the less they're able to help other people cope with the problem.

I play darts occasionally and if I'm lucky I can walk around the room. That's about all the exercise I can manage. I have realized that for somebody with M.E., walking up and down stairs, drying your hair, washing yourself, drying yourself, cooking a meal, is exercise in itself. It varies from case to case.

I've had few holidays since the M.E. began. I used to go on a lot of walking holidays but that was mainly because my husband liked them. I don't know what I would have done if he hadn't been so keen on walking. I've never been a beach and sun person but now of course it would make me ill in any case. I suppose I have this nice fantasy of being on a beautiful Scottish island somewhere and writing a book, that's the kind of holiday I'd like to have. If you start thinking about organizing a holiday, you'd never get there.

I go to Guernsey because it's a small place. It's easy to drive round and there's lots to see. I've got friends there now and it isn't far to fly. I'm not someone who hates being at home or being inside. Stephen Fry was interviewed the other day on 'Sunday Night Clive' and he said that he would as soon draw his curtains and sit by a nice warm fire. I've a lot of sympathy with that. I'm lucky, I live somewhere with a beautiful view outside my window, so I don't miss holidays terribly. I'd love to go to Ireland again but I would need someone with me. I'd go if I had a companion who'd do the driving and be responsible if something goes wrong.

I was invited by someone to go up to one of the islands in Scotland to do a lecture on M.E. It's not just the travelling or the cost of getting there that's difficult, it's needing someone to travel with me. If I was fit I would go like a shot. If they could 'beam me up, Scottie', I'd be there.

I do suffer from memory loss. I've forgotten how much I suffer from it. Sometimes I don't even know what I've forgotten. It's not as bad now as it was but I have trouble recalling things – people's names, for example.

Darrell Ho-Yen stated in his book that women find sex more difficult than men when they've got M.E. I said to him that's a lot of nonsense. It's easier for a woman, at least she can lie back and think of England. We had a laugh about it, but what he really meant was that women seem to need more counselling. It may be that when you've got M.E. you have to be able to say I can only manage this or that, and I'd like to do the other but I'm not fit enough at the moment, and so on. I think women feel guilty about not being able to please. Perhaps they feel their role is to satisfy their male counterparts. Men have always been quite happy to say what they want, or if they are too tired to do anything. From what Dr Ho-Yen was saying they don't seem to feel the guilt that women get bogged down with.

There are practical problems, things like aches and pains and tenderness. The worst is the lack of energy, palpitations, feeling breathless. You have to experiment with different positions and not be embarrassed about doing something you might not have done otherwise. There's still such a taboo regarding masturbation, for instance, but in fact it's such a helpful, useful thing. I talked about masturbation with Dr Ho-Yen, and he said that if a woman is in too much pain inside, then perhaps she could masturbate the man. I said, 'Are you joking? You haven't a clue about M.E. Unless he's going to come in thirty seconds you'd not be able to manage that!'

The first thing to consider is keeping your heart rate down and just to have a really enjoyable time. Which is possible if you can relax. You have to learn to give and take pleasure in different ways and that's what it's all about. I think in some ways it's liberating because you probably have to think about things that able-bodied people don't. It makes you more inventive. When people are really, really ill in the early stages of M.E. they couldn't have a sexual relationship. But later on, there are days when you have more energy, if you time it just right.

# Caroline Abrehart

Caroline is sixteen, a part-time student, who has had M.E. for four years and is making a slow recovery. She lives in South Devon.

It started about four years ago when I was twelve. First of all I had a pain in my back and the doctor told me it was growing pains. It got much worse, and he gave me some exercises to do every hour which was the worst possible thing he could have suggested. It began in my lower back, spread up my spine and into my shoulders and neck and down my arms and legs. I got weaker and weaker. I had come down with a virus at the time and my back was so bad I couldn't sit, and had to lie down. My doctor sent me for an x-ray and to a specialist; he found it really difficult to believe. He basically ridiculed me. Then I saw a paediatrician and he told me, after lots of blood tests, that he was about 98 percent sure that I had post-viral fatigue syndrome. He didn't say M.E. We were pretty happy to have it diagnosed, as before that we just didn't have a clue what it could be and it was really frightening not knowing. Then I went to see a rheumatologist. He thought it was spondylitis, and gave me some anti-inflammatory tablets, saying that I'd feel better in a couple of days. I didn't. The next time I went back he told me that I had juvenile arthritis, and just gave me something to take the pain away. The time after that it was a very rare form of arthritis. When I went back to the paediatrician and the rheumatologist, they told me that it was psychological and I was sent to a psychiatric nurse. He asked me questions like, 'Which parent do you like best?' and things like that, suggesting in a way that I was school-phobic. Just about everything I told him, he twisted round, and I actually felt that I was on trial, as if I'd done something wrong.

During that stage I was spending all of my time in bed. I occasionally got up for a meal on a good day, and it was terrible because I had to sit around for hours in waiting rooms to see these people. By the time I got in there I was in such a daze that I could hardly hear what they were saying to me. Then I just decided that I wasn't going to see anybody else. I was pretty sure that I had M.E., and I'd talked to a friend who had it. My GP was quite helpful as well, and he thought that I had M.E. We heard about a private doctor in Ivybridge, and as the school doctor had been very unhelpful, we went to see Dr West. She was the first person who actually knew how I felt. She said, 'I bet you feel really exhausted and can't stand up for too long.' She actually understood the problems that I had, and she said that I definitely had M.E. She did a few tests and she told me that I was allergic to wheat and dairy products and that I had candida. I gradually came off dairy products, sugar and wheat, and then she gave me vitamin and mineral supplements. I had to go to Dr Betty Dowsett because the school doctor wanted a second opinion. Dr Dowsett said that I was doing everything right, and to carry on. I started aromatherapy which was very helpful because I was so puffy and my skin was tender to the touch; my lymphatic system wasn't working properly through lack of exercise. I made quite good progress, it was really helpful because I was still getting quite severe backache and nerve pains (which were helped by magnesium). I'm still having aromatherapy for my back and cranio-sacral therapy, and I find that sticking to a strict diet and making sure I rest when I need to is important.

Last year was the first year that I attended school regularly again. I didn't go very much when I didn't know what was wrong with me. I was going in for a few days and then being ill. It was very difficult because everyone was asking me what was wrong and every time I went in I had something different to say, it was really very awkward. I only took one GCSE, English, so I did miss the lot, but I am catching up and I will do them. Now I'm back at school studying French GCSE. I'm also studying maths privately to take my GCSE, as I missed about three years of this, and I'm taking my English A Level. I was hoping to take French A Level which I'd always planned to do as it's my best subject, but I feel that I've just missed too much. I don't think I'm going to be able to do it. I'd like to go to university; I'm interested in English literature. I'm not entirely sure what after that, though. I'm quite interested in the media.

I'm an optimistic person, and I believe that I've got to learn from being ill and once you've learnt all you can from that, then it's time to be well again. Being ill has taught me to change my lifestyle for the better. I've had a lot of time to look at myself. I think I'm definitely a lot more in touch with who I am, I know myself a lot better. I was pretty silly before. I think you have to become more mature. I certainly found when I came back from meeting people after contracting M.E. that I felt a bit more mature than them. I felt more serious than them, that I knew what I wanted and would work, for instance, in school when they were messing around. I wanted to get things done because I wanted to get somewhere and I felt that I'd wasted enough time already. I just wanted to get on with things. If I saw people wasting what they had, you know, not doing anything with their life, that made me really angry. I was a really ambitious sort of person, and I found it hard to have to sit back and watch people squander their opportunities.

I think I've also become a lot more sensitive to other people. I've certainly gained patience which you really have to have with M.E. When I was really ill I found that I was very, very aware of the feelings of people around me and I took these on in a way. I found that I was taking on people's problems, but now I can get on with that a lot better. I think having M.E. makes you very sensitive to everything, not only different kinds of pain.

I wouldn't want to go back and not have the experience of M.E. I wouldn't want to go back to the person I was before. I've also made some really good friends, and I now have some very strong friendships. But it's a scary thing to have a long illness. I really felt that I was missing out on things. I was a very sporty person, I did a lot of sport, and I had to give all that up.

I played hockey and netball for the school team, and tennis, and I used to do a lot of horse-riding. I worked at the stables all Sunday, which was very hard work, and I had to give that up as well. So I experienced a real sense of isolation, and I still feel quite isolated sometimes. I spent the first couple of years completely cut off from people; I couldn't do anything at all during that time. It's quite difficult even now, because I can go out with my friends but I can only do so much. It's really holding me back a lot at the moment. I can't go out and feel well and it affects my moods. I've found that if I go out and I'm not feeling that well, then I just want to sit in a corner, which makes me feel completely hideous and very heavy, and that's not what I feel I should be feeling. It should be a time for me to go out and enjoy myself, go to parties and things; I can deal with just being tired, but being in pain and tired makes it very hard to be sociable and a normal person.

On the positive side, I think you learn to value things more. The things that I can do now have become incredibly important to me, whereas before I just took them for granted. I have some great friends who've really stuck by me, and I think that I value the things that I can do much more than normal people. But I do feel I've missed out – if I go to a school play or something, for example. I love drama, and I was totally missing out on that and it really depressed me. It was all right being at home because for a while I was just too tired to think about anything else, my world was my bedroom. But after I came out of that I became much more aware of what I was missing out on – and I still am. I couldn't see the positive side of things because all I could see was how unfair it was, and how all my friends seemed to get on with their lives.

I felt very angry for a long time. I was in pain all the time and I wasn't sleeping and I just didn't know what was happening to me. To be told by various doctors that what was actually happening couldn't really be happening, and that I couldn't really be feeling like that, made me very angry. And very confused. You always expect when you're younger to go to the doctor and for them to give you something that makes you better. You don't expect to be told that you're not feeling what you're feeling. I also found it very difficult because I was in such a vulnerable position. To actually speak up, and say, 'Well hang on, listen to me', was difficult. I was supposed to be a child, they were supposed to be the adults, and I wasn't supposed to know better than them. I found that very much with the school doctor. I felt I knew what I needed to do and how I needed to look after myself, and she was telling my parents that they were supposed to be forcing me to go back to school because that's what I really needed. I was saying, no, it's not, and she couldn't accept that a thirteen-year-old knew better than she did. That was very awkward. In the end I did speak up for myself because I just got so fed up with being spoken down to. I had to say I haven't done anything wrong, and I feel like you're accusing me of something.

Lately, what's been really satisfying is getting back into the social world again. I was very worried at one time that I wasn't going to be able to go back to school and take up where I left off, because people were saying, 'Well, what have you been doing then?' and I'd say, 'Lying in bed, just being sick.' I thought it was going to be so hard to be accepted, but what's been most satisfying is that I've made a lot more friends. I have been going out a lot and *managing* to do things and meet people. If there's something I really want to do, if I really want to go to see a group or something, then I'll kind of look after myself for the week beforehand and kind of build up to it. Other people might go out every night in the holidays, but I have to build up to one night that's really important to me, and then I make sure I really enjoy it.

I find that I get really enthusiastic about things, I'm a very enthusiastic person. Listening to music is therapeutic for me because I feel that I can get everything out of my system. I hate rave bands, dance stuff with no meaning. I like intense sort of stuff, energetic. I like passionate music. I used to play the piano but gave that up when my hands became painful.

There have been unexpected things about being ill. But then it's hard to know what to expect really, because when I first got M.E. I didn't know what it was and so there was a lot of reading up to do. I had to learn about pain quite a lot; before, I think I was always pretty wet about pain. You know, if I fell over or something I'd make a real fuss, but I had to learn to live with being in pain and just to cope with it. I think that's quite an important thing. I got very sharp pains that I couldn't put down to anything. From doing nothing, just all of a sudden they'd stab me in the chest, and that would be quite scary. Now I just think, oh right, and get on with it. Quite recently I've had heart palpitations in school where my heart's racing, and I think I'm going to pass out. Things seem to come on for no apparent reason, and that's frightening.

People often think I'm drunk, which is quite funny. I tend to go down to the pub with my friends when we meet, and I'm completely teetotal, but people often think I'm completely drunk. My balance is not always very good, especially if I'm tired, so I kind of stagger around. Often people look because I just stare into space quite happily when I get tired. I have been asked if I'm on drugs. I have walked into lamp-posts before, just from not quite being aware of what's going on around me. And looking back, seeing the psychiatric nurse was quite funny because it's just so ridiculous. He seemed to think that I'd been abused or something. At the time, though, it upset me.

Since having M.E. I think I've learnt a lot about control, because I used to be a chocaholic. I'm on a very, very strict diet at the moment. I don't eat dairy products, wheat, sugar or meat. I don't even find that I can replace sugar with things like apples because they happen to be bad for my candida, so I don't really have anything like that. Sometimes I'd like to eat fruit, so I've had to learn to be especially strict. I think I have learnt self-discipline. But it's difficult because it is tempting to rush things.

I started riding about a year and a half ago. I actually got back to where I was galloping along, and then I fell off, quite badly, which was the worst possible thing to do. I find I'm incredibly sensitive to touch, and if I bash myself then it really hurts, so falling off a horse at a gallop really put me back. But I was enjoying that, I did manage to do it and I expect I will again when I'm up to it.

Going back to school was very difficult because I had not really seen anybody. I'd lost touch with people, all my friends from school, I just hadn't been able to see them, and I felt that I was under pressure to go back when I wasn't ready. I felt I had to take on a lot of responsibility at a young age. I was having to decide when I was ready to go back to school and whether it was that I didn't feel well enough to go back or whether it was that I just couldn't face it. I did want to go back, the problem was that the getting back was awesome.

I felt like I was in a bubble. I felt very separate from everybody else and all the noise and everything. I just didn't know whether I could cope and I had to really trust myself. Then I found, and I still find, that if I don't want to go to school it's usually because I'm just not up to it. When I am feeling up to it, I really do want to be in school. I have to trust myself and say well that is OK, instead of forcing myself. People always say, 'Well, do you think you could just kind of try?' and I say, 'Well, no, I really don't feel ready yet.' I actually made the decision to go back and see my home tutor in school instead of out of school. She is very supportive, a lovely person, who has really helped me get back. I found that walking down the corridors made me feel isolated, even though there were people all around me. I felt completely separate from everybody else, and I just didn't feel I fitted in at all. I was going in for my English lessons every day. I was seeing people in class, but not at break times, and I found that once I started going in at break time, I was kind of on the edge of conversations because I didn't feel that I was up to making small talk. I hadn't been out and done really exciting things, and I felt talking about M.E. was really boring for people.

People do discriminate against you. It's the people like doctors who don't understand, and just tell you that you can't be feeling what you are feeling, that's the main sort of discrimination. In school, most of the teachers were very helpful but some just couldn't understand certain aspects of M.E. I got the impression from some that they thought that if I tried really hard, then I could do things. I had to try and explain to them that I couldn't, that I really did want to do them, it wasn't just because I was lazy.

Other pupils gave me stick too to begin with. They called me a skiver. They'd ask, 'How's your back, then?' and I'd say, 'Well, actually, it's not just my back,' but they didn't understand any of it, because I didn't understand it. I remember going in one day for a math's class, which was all I went in for for about a couple of weeks, and a girl, whom I didn't get on with particularly well, said, 'Why do you bother just coming in for one class, why don't you just stop, why just one class?' I was so surprised, I didn't know what to say. I'd been lying in bed for the last couple of months and hadn't seen anybody, and I just didn't want to lose contact with the outside world. That's why I was coming in for a tiny amount of time, just because it was important to stay in touch with people, to carry on and try and be slightly normal.

Of course I looked normal most of the time. It was only after I'd been away from school for a couple of years, other pupils began to realize that there was something actually wrong. I think there was a bit of jealousy in a way from people who didn't want to be in school. They thought that I was having a great time, and that I could watch videos and television all day. Later they actually became quite interested in my condition.

At the beginning of the illness I thought I was going to die, so I didn't believe I was going to be able to do anything; *anything* after that was an achievement really. Starting riding again was quite good, and I went to see the Levellers last year. I never thought I'd go to a concert again, and that was standing as well; it was an amazing achievement for me. As was taking my English GCSE.

Of course, I've had failures too. I tried to play tennis with my Dad, which was really, really stupid. It was quite early on in the illness and I was feeling quite good and I just hate being unfit. It was a really nice day and Dad said, 'Why don't we have a game of tennis?' We ended up playing for about three-quarters of an hour, having quite a good game of tennis, and then I just kind of collapsed. I wasn't very experienced in managing my illness then. There were also certain subjects at school that I had difficulties with. I found maths a real struggle because I just couldn't make connections in my head, so I just gave that up for a while. I got so frustrated. I found that sometimes I'd actually forget what I was saying half way through a sentence, and I did that when I was writing as well. I'd be writing away and suddenly I'd wonder what was I saying and have to actually read over what I'd written.

Perhaps I should give a checklist of my symptoms. I had lots of different kinds of pain. I had nerve pain, joint pain and muscle pain, my muscles went into spasm quite a lot. I wasn't really affected by headaches like a lot of people, so that was OK. My temperature was weird, my friends around me said I was really contrary because when everyone else was warm, I was cold, and vice versa. I get so many symptoms, it's hard to explain. I have just about every stomach problem, and I find that because I have been in bed for so long my lymphatic system doesn't work very well. I find that I'm quite sensitive to touch, and have quite a lot of swelling so sometimes even my clothes hurt me. I have brain symptoms too: my short-term memory is not brilliant.

There are things I think I'll never do again. I can't imagine playing hockey for the life of me, partly because my back is still quite bad. I can't imagine bending over and running. Maybe I'll be able to get back to it but I can't really see that happening. As for going to a football match and things like that, they won't be impossible in the future but for the time being they are out of the question. I have got to the stage where I can take some gentle exercise. I'm actually starting yoga soon, and I'm hoping that will be helpful. I feel that I'm at the stage where my muscles are so weak that they need to be built up, but it's got to be at the right time, I've got to be well enough to do it. I don't believe in telling people with M.E. that they should be exercising because they've been in bed for too long. It's got to be the right time, otherwise it could be damaging.

We haven't been abroad for quite a long time. I went to Paris with my Dad and my brother when I was first having back pains. It was actually in Paris when it first started, I remember, which must have been about four years ago. We went up to York for a week last year, and that was really good because everywhere was within walking distance. We stayed in a flat that was near the centre so there were lots of things to do. It was nice to get away and have a break, and we're hoping to go away this year.

I don't have a boyfriend. I've found that that was totally impossible to even think about because I just wasn't seeing people, and now I feel that having M.E. inhibits me a lot. I don't suppose having M.E. would be a problem physically, it's more how it affects me mentally. I mean, recently I've been tired a lot, and I find when I go out and see people that I just don't have the confidence to be really sociable, and it makes me feel unattractive. I feel that that's really inhibiting.

I think I've changed my friends. A few of them didn't stick by me very well, and weren't very supportive, but I had two very good friends who have stuck by me and now I'm a lot closer to them because of that. They're very good, they won't let me overdo things and say, 'I think you ought to have a lie-down now.' They've been through it with me, they understand, and they want to know about it. When I do go out they've seen me in a really bad state and they've been with me in school when I've had things like heart palpitations. They've held my hand, and they're getting very good at sorting me out and knowing what to do in difficult situations.

It was very hard with my parents too to start off with. I felt really guilty because they were so worried about me. I got more and more withdrawn and I saw them getting more and more worried, and I felt that I ought to be kind of doing things to show them that I was all right but I couldn't. Mum got quite depressed because she just couldn't help me, and she's always been there to pick me up and set me on my feet. But she couldn't do anything and I saw how hard it was for her, more so than my father because it was Mum who I was spending much more time with as Dad was at work. I could see how my being ill really affected her life and how it made everything more difficult for her. She couldn't do a lot of things that she wanted to do and that made me feel really responsible.

Being so close to each other and with each other, without being able to get away from each other all the time, I was very aware of how she felt. When she was depressed I felt terrible, because I felt that it was my fault. Very often we'd end up arguing over stupid things. I couldn't get out of the house and if I got frustrated I couldn't go out for a run like my Dad probably would, or go out for a drive, or even walk or whatever. I was so dependent on my parents because I couldn't really do much for myself at all, and I felt that I was holding them back.

I have a brother and he and I have become a lot closer in the last year, probably because we've grown up quite a lot. We go out together sometimes with a few friends which we wouldn't have done before. It's mostly that I have taken centre stage – so everything has to revolve around me. My brother has to walk the dog all the time, that's just a small example but he's had to take on things like that. I don't think he's particularly resentful of it though. We can talk to each other quite a lot. When we first started really talking to each other, it was when I'd thrown a complete wobbly because I was very, very frustrated. He helped me to understand that. He could kind of see that if he was missing out on all the things that I was at my age, he would feel the same way.

At school my teachers are now all really good about it. If I want to put my head down on the desk and go to sleep, then that's fine, they all accept that. I have set myself very high standards at school, and that's my problem. One of the hardest things was to accept that, well, maybe I'll only get a low grade in this one whereas before I would have got a good mark. I find that a difficult compromise, to just get through it instead of doing really well, I don't like it at all. As a result I put more pressure on myself than anyone else does. They would say, 'Oh well, hand it in whenever you like,' but I want to be the normal one, and I want to get things done on time, no matter what. But I'm learning to relax a bit, and to appreciate that sticking to a strict timetable is not the most important thing.

My GP is very sympathetic. He'll prescribe anything that I want to try, but he doesn't really suggest anything because he doesn't really know an awful lot about M.E. That's good, because he's not pretending that he does, but he's not dismissive of it either. I found the school doctor extremely unhelpful. I remember she came to see me when I was in bed, and she wouldn't look me in the eye while she was talking to me. I was trying to explain to her how I felt and then she told Mum that she thought I should go back to school. I just felt that she had turned everything that she'd heard around to suit her own diagnosis, instead of actually hearing what I was saying in context. Mum was telling her about what Dr West had done, which was to take my blood pressure when I was lying down and then when I was standing up, and how it actually dropped when I stood up instead of rising. The school doctor seemed to imply that it was somatic, that is, a psychological problem. Dr West, the clinical ecologist at Ivybridge, had taken my pulse too and found that it was racing all the time. The school doctor said that was psychological as well.

The most difficult thing about seeing different doctors was that they all said different things. I'd got used to thinking that I had post-viral fatigue syndrome; I had read up a lot on M.E., and it seemed likely. Once I had accepted that I had it, for them then to take that back and say, 'Oh well, actually, it's all in your mind,' was really very cruel.

I have found that of all the treatments I've tried, the alternative treatments have helped most. First of all I saw a reflexologist, and I found that incredibly painful. I couldn't really cope because I was very sensitive to touch. It was just too much for me, so I kind of gave up on that. Then I saw the aromatherapist. She's been very, very helpful, she's like my counsellor and we talk about everything. I find that she understands me and wants to understand the illness, unlike doctors who reject what I tell them. With her I felt that I managed to kind of clear up what was in my head a bit more. I felt that was part of what was isolating me, that I was having to deal with a lot of extra things myself. I still see her as well as a herbalist. The herbalist's helped quite a lot too – not cured me, but I have improved.

The various different alternative treatments have all helped in their different ways. They've all helped at different stages of the illness. The aromatherapist helped me first of all with the puffiness and the lymphatic problems; the cranio-sacral therapist helped me with my back problems. Dr West, the clinical ecologist, did all kinds of tests – kinesiology tests for mineral and vitamin deficiencies, and a test for allergies. They complement each other; they are also sympathetic, caring sort of people who actually want to help you. Their kind of attention is so much better than being rushed into a poky little room for five minutes, after sitting outside for an hour and a half, to be told you're out of your mind by someone who looks as though he needs a psychiatrist more than you do.

I think most things on the National Health, apart from my GP who prescribed the minerals and vitamins that I need, have been very unhelpful. I would like to see GPs educated about M.E. I think they should be taught in a different way so that they are more open-minded. Just because they don't recognize something as being in their text book doesn't mean it doesn't exist. If you don't fit into a certain section, then you don't get any help at all. I think that that ought to be changed. I don't really know enough about medical schools but I certainly think that things like M.E. ought to be brought into the syllabus or whatever. The medical profession generally must be made aware of the problems that people with M.E. have experienced at the hands of doctors who don't recognize the disease, and MS too in the early stages. Doctors must be made aware of environmental things like the organo-phosphates that are sprayed on things and in the water, because I'm sure this has an effect on M.E. sufferers. A lot of farmers spray the crops round here and I know that the symptoms that farmers have got from organo-phosphate poisoning are quite similar to M.E. There are chemicals in everything – it's quite frightening. Even paint or perfume just knock me out completely. We did a touch of painting in the house quite early on in my illness which triggered a complete relapse for me. Perfume samples in magazines – people are unaware of the effect they can have. I think that doctors should be made much more aware of things like that, and the side effects of drugs.

One thing that has affected me very badly is painkillers. I was taking eight co-drydromol a day, which are quite strong painkillers, that the doctor prescribed for me but I wasn't told anything about their side effects. When I stopped taking those, I was taking eight paracetamol a day. With my memory lapses I forget how many I take, and I'm sure I've taken too many, and they have damaged my liver. My liver isn't right at all at the moment, and I still haven't managed to sort it out. I thought I needed painkillers to keep me well, and wasn't told how they could affect me. They didn't really help the pain, either, for once I stopped taking them the pain didn't get any worse.

Action for M.E. do a really good job making people aware, but I think it's important to get people to be *interested* in M.E. and to be curious about it. I think this yuppie flu thing the media have latched on to would be dismissed if people actually tried to understand what it's all about instead of just stereotyping people.

I think it's really important to get in touch with other people with M.E. just so that you don't feel so alone. You can feel really cut off, that you're the only one who feels like this. You must not give up hope of getting better, because you *can* recover, and you must be able to believe in yourself. I think it's really important to have things like support groups – that's what people need, a sympathetic ear.

You shouldn't believe everything that doctors tell you and take it as gospel. Too many people think, 'Oh well, if the doctor says that, then it must be true,' but it's not. You have to try and get in touch with yourself a bit more and try and find out what's going on with yourself rather than just believing someone who doesn't really have a clue.

# Recommended Further Reading

Collinge, William:    *Recovering from M.E., A Guide to Self Empowerment* (Souvenir Press)
Ho-Yen, Dr Darrell:   *Better Recovery from Viral Illnesses* (Dodona Books)
MacIntyre, Dr Anne:   *Postviral Fatigue Syndrome, How to Live with it* (Thorsons)
Shepherd, Dr Charles: *Living with M.E.* (Mandarin)

If you would like to know more about M.E., you may wish to contact the following:

**Action for M.E.**
P.O. Box 1302
Wells
BA5 2WE
Tel: (01749) 670799
Fax: (01749) 679193

Action for M.E. is a national charitable trust which provides information and support services to people with M.E., their families, friends and carers, and funds research and campaigns to change attitudes towards the disease. Action for M.E. supports a network of over 200 groups and contacts throughout the United Kingdom and publishes a journal (*Interaction*) and factsheets on M.E. and available therapies, as well as advice sheets for doctors, employers, young people and their carers.

# Other titles in this series available from Boxtree

*Link to Life: Spinal Cord Injury*
Contributing Editor: Lydia Thomas

*Link to Life: Epilepsy*
Contributing Editor: Gary Johnstone
(published March 1995)

These books are available from your local bookshop or newsagent, or can
be ordered by credit card on the following number: 01903 732596

Alternatively, complete the following order form and return to:

Littlehampton Book Services
14 Eldon Way
Lineside Industrial Estate
Littlehampton
West Sussex BN17 7EH

------------------------------------------------------------------------

Please supply the following titles:

I enclose a cheque for £ ..................... + £1.00 postage and packing made
payable to Littlehampton Book Services.

| Quantity | Title | ISBN | Price |
|---|---|---|---|
| ............... | Spinal Cord Injury | 1 85283 9058 | £6.99 |
| ............... | Epilepsy | 1 85283 9285 | £6.99 |

Name: . . . . . . . . . . . . . . . . . . . . . . . . . . . . . . . . . . . . .

Address: . . . . . . . . . . . . . . . . . . . . . . . . . . . . . . . . . . . .

. . . . . . . . . . . . . . . . . . . . . . . . . . . . . . . . . . . .

Postcode: . . . . . . . . . . . . . . . . . . . . . .

Tel: . . . . . . . . . . . . . . . . . . . . . . .